T0255727

# GI Emergencies
## A Quick Reference Guide

# GI Emergencies
## A Quick Reference Guide

Edited by:

*Robert C. Lowe, MD*
*Education Director, Section of Gastroenterology*
*Boston Medical Center*
*Associate Professor of Medicine*
*Boston University School of Medicine*
*Boston, Massachusetts*

*Francis A. Farraye, MD, MSc*
*Clinical Director, Section of Gastroenterology*
*Boston Medical Center*
*Professor of Medicine*
*Boston University School of Medicine*
*Boston, Massachusetts*

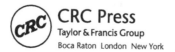

**CRC Press**
Taylor & Francis Group
Boca Raton   London   New York

CRC Press is an imprint of the
Taylor & Francis Group, an **informa** business

First published 2012 by SLACK Incorporated

Published 2024 by CRC Press
2385 NW Executive Center Drive, Suite 320, Boca Raton FL 33431

and by CRC Press
4 Park Square, Milton Park, Abingdon, Oxon, OX14 4RN

*CRC Press is an imprint of Taylor & Francis Group, LLC*

Library of Congress Cataloging-in-Publication Data

GI emergencies : a quick reference guide / edited by Robert C. Lowe, Francis A. Farraye.
    p. ; cm.
  Includes bibliographical references and index.
  ISBN 978-1-55642-990-3 (pbk. : alk. paper)  1. Gastrointestinal system--Diseases--Case studies. 2. Gastrointestinal system--Diseases--Handbooks, manuals, etc. 3. Gastrointestinal emergencies--Case studies. 4. Gastrointestinal emergencies--Handbooks, manuals, etc. I. Lowe, Robert C., 1966- II. Farraye, Francis A.
  [DNLM: 1. Gastrointestinal Diseases--diagnosis--Case Reports. 2. Gastrointestinal Diseases--diagnosis--Handbooks. 3. Gastrointestinal Diseases--therapy--Case Reports. 4. Gastrointestinal Diseases--therapy--Handbooks. 5. Emergencies--Case Reports. 6. Emergencies--Handbooks. 7. Evidence-Based Medicine--Case Reports. 8. Evidence-Based Medicine--Handbooks. WI 39]
  RC808.G67 2011
  616.3'3--dc23
                                    2011021738

ISBN: 9781556429903 (pbk)
ISBN: 9781003524366 (ebk)

DOI: 10.1201/9781003524366

# Dedication

I dedicate this book to the medical students, residents, and GI fellows that I have worked with over the years; their curiosity and love of medicine has made my work as a clinical educator joyful and rewarding. I further dedicate this textbook to my wife, Amy, and my children, Katherine and David, who have made my life richer through their love and support.

*Robert C. Lowe, MD*

This book is written for all the medical students, house staff, and gastroenterology fellows that I have had the opportunity to work with during the past 20 years. It is my hope that they learned as much from me as I have from them. This book is further dedicated to my loving and devoted family: my wife, Renee M. Remily, MD; my children, Jennifer and Alexis Farraye; and my parents, who taught me that hard work, perseverance, and commitment can result in great accomplishments.

*Francis A. Farraye, MD, MSc*

# CONTENTS

# ACKNOWLEDGMENTS

We would like to thank the authors for their excellent contributions. The combined effort of trainees and experienced faculty members has created a novel educational tool that will be of use to practitioners at all levels of training. We would also like to thank the team at SLACK Incorporated, especially Carrie Kotlar, who appreciated the importance of this work and guided us in the production of this textbook.

# ABOUT THE EDITORS

*Robert C. Lowe, MD* is an associate professor of medicine at the Boston University School of Medicine (BUSM) in Massachusetts and is the Fellowship Director for the Section of Gastroenterology at Boston Medical Center (BMC). Dr. Lowe received his BA from Harvard College, Cambridge, Massachusetts, in 1988 and his MD from Harvard Medical School in 1992. He completed his internal medicine residency at the Brigham and Women's Hospital in Boston, where he was selected to be Chief Medical Resident. He trained in gastroenterology at BMC and has been on staff at BMC since 2001. His clinical interests include general gastroenterology and hepatology, with a particular interest in the care of patients with viral liver diseases and cirrhosis.

Dr. Lowe is also heavily involved with the educational program at Boston University and BMC. In addition to his work as Fellowship Director for the Section of Gastroenterology, he is a dedicated Educator in the BMC Department of Medicine, attending several months each year on the medicine wards and facilitating a bimonthly educational conference for house staff. At BUSM, he is the Director of the Second Year Vision Committee, which administers an integrated preclinical course for the entire second-year class; he also serves as the course director for the gastroenterology module. He serves on the school's Medical Education Committee, the governing body at BUSM for curriculum and educational planning and oversight. He is active in curriculum development for medical students, house officers, and fellows and is particularly involved in the teaching of clinical reasoning skills and the fostering of professionalism among medical trainees.

Dr. Lowe is the recipient of multiple teaching awards and was recently designated one of the "Best of Boston" by *Boston* magazine. He is the author of numerous book chapters and review articles, and he is co-editor of the *Educational Review Manual in Gastroenterology*. For the past 4 years, he has served as the chairman of the Medical Advisory Committee of the American Liver Foundation, New England Chapter, and he serves as a member of the AGA Education and Training Committee, which began in June 2011.

*Francis A. Farraye, MD, MSc* is Professor of Medicine at the Boston University School of Medicine. He is also Clinical Director in the Section of Gastroenterology and Co-Director of the Center for Digestive Disorders at Boston Medical Center. After graduating from the State University of New York at Stony Brook, Dr. Farraye earned his medical doctorate from the Albert Einstein College of Medicine in Bronx, New York and his master's degree in epidemiology from the Harvard School of Public Health in Boston. He completed an internal medicine residency and gastroenterology fellowship at the Beth Israel Hospital in Boston.

Dr. Farraye's clinical interests are in the care of patients with inflammatory bowel disease and the management of colon polyps and colorectal cancer. He is studying vitamin D absorption in patients with inflammatory bowel disease, the management and diagnosis of dysplasia and cancer in patients with inflammatory bowel disease, and predictors of pouch complications after ileal pouch anal anastomosis. In the area of colorectal cancer, he is examining the role of hyperplastic polyps as an alternative pathway in the development of colorectal cancer.

A frequent speaker and invited lecturer on topics on the diagnosis and management of inflammatory bowel disease, Dr. Farraye has authored or co-authored more than 250 original scientific manuscripts, chapters, reviews, and abstracts. He is co-editor of the text *Bariatric Surgery: A Primer for Your Medical Practice;* associate editor for *Therapy for Digestive Disorders;* series editor for *Curbside Consultation in Gastroenterology;* and co-editor of the text *Curbside Consultation in IBD.* His most recent book for patients is *Questions and Answers About Ulcerative Colitis.*

Dr. Farraye is a fellow of the American College of Physicians, American Society of Gastrointestinal Endoscopy (ASGE), American Gastroenterological Association (AGA), and the American College of Gastroenterology (ACG). He has served as the AGA representative on the National Colorectal Cancer Round Table, chair of the lower gastrointestinal disorders section of the Annual Scientific Program Committee of the ASGE, and a member of the ASGE Technology Committee. Nationally, he is a member of the Board of Trustees in the ACG, Crohn's and Colitis Foundation of America (CCFA), Professional Education Committee and the Chapter Medical Advisory Committee for the New England CCFA, as well as a past chairman. The New England CCFA named Dr. Farraye Humanitarian of the Year in 2003. He was the 2009 recipient of the ACG William Carey Award for service to the college. Dr. Farraye was listed as a "Best of Boston" gastroenterologist in 2010.

# CONTRIBUTING AUTHORS

*Uri Avissar, MD (Chapter 2)*
Assistant Professor of Medicine
Boston University School of Medicine
Section of Gastroenterology
Boston Medical Center
Boston, Massachusetts

*Wanda P. Blanton, MD (Chapter 5)*
Instructor in Medicine
Division of Gastroenterology and Hepatology
Boston University School of Medicine
Boston, Massachusetts

*Charles M. Bliss Jr., MD, FACP (Chapter 12)*
Clinical Assistant Professor of Medicine
Boston University School of Medicine
Section of Gastroenterology
Boston Medical Center
Boston, Massachusetts

*Audrey H. Calderwood, MD (Chapter 3)*
Assistant Professor of Medicine
Boston University School of Medicine
Section of Gastroenterology
Boston, Massachusetts

*Joseph Feuerstein, MD (Chapter 4)*
Gastroenterology Fellow
Division of Gastroenterology
Beth Israel Deaconess Medical Center
Boston, Massachusetts

*Stephen D. Humm, MD (Chapter 8)*
Gastroenterology Fellow
Boston University School of Medicine
Section of Gastroenterology
Boston Medical Center
Boston, Massachusetts

*Christopher S. Huang, MD (Chapter 8)*
Assistant Professor of Medicine
Boston University School of Medicine
Section of Gastroenterology
Boston Medical Center
Boston, Massachusetts

*Sujai Jalaj, MD (Chapter 11)*
Internal Medicine Resident
Department of Internal Medicine
Boston University Medical Center
Boston, Massachusetts

*Aarti Kakkar, MD (Chapter 10)*
Gastroenterology Fellow
Section of Gastroenterology
Boston Medical Center
Boston, Massachusetts

*Joann Kwah, MD (Chapter 5)*
Gastroenterology Fellow
Division of Gastroenterology and Hepatology
Boston Medical Center
Boston, Massachusetts

*David R. Lichtenstein, MD (Chapter 7)*
Director of Endoscopy
Associate Professor of Medicine
Boston University School of Medicine
Section of Gastroenterology
Boston Medical Center
Boston, Massachusetts

*Caroline Loeser, MD (Chapter 13)*
Assistant Professor of Medicine
Boston University School of Medicine
Section of Gastroenterology
Boston Medical Center
Boston, Massachusetts

*Daniel S. Mishkin, MD, CM, FRCP(C) (Chapter 11)*
Assistant Professor of Medicine
Boston University School of Medicine
Boston, Massachusetts

*David P. Nunes, MD (Chapter 10)*
Associate Professor of Medicine
Boston University School of Medicine
Section of Gastroenterology
Boston Medical Center
Boston, Massachusetts

*Marcos C. Pedrosa, MD, MPH (Chapter 1)*
Associate Professor of Medicine
Boston University School of Medicine
Gastroenterology Section
VA Boston Healthcare System
Boston, Massachusetts

*Rajeev Prabakaran, MD (Chapter 9)*
Gastroenterology Fellow
Boston University School of Medicine
Section of Gastroenterology
Boston Medical Center
Boston, Massachusetts

*Ivonne Ramirez, MD (Chapter 7)*
Gastroenterology Fellow
Section of Gastroenterology
Boston Medical Center
Boston, Massachusetts

*Ashraf Saleemuddin, MD (Chapter 2)*
Gastroenterology Fellow
Boston University School of Medicine
Section of Gastroenterology
Boston Medical Center
Boston, Massachusetts

*Jennifer A. Sinclair, MD (Chapters 12, 13)*
Gastroenterology Fellow
Boston University School of Medicine
Section of Gastroenterology
Boston Medical Center
Boston, Massachusetts

*Pushpak Taunk, MD (Chapter 1)*
Gastroenterology Fellow
Section of Gastroenterology
Boston University School of Medicine
Boston, Massachusetts

*Hillary Tompkins, MD (Chapter 3)*
Gastroenterology Fellow
Department of Medicine
Boston Medical Center
Boston, Massachusetts

*Sharmeel K. Wasan, MD (Chapter 6)*
Assistant Professor of Medicine
Boston University School of Medicine
Section of Gastroenterology
Boston Medical Center
Boston, Massachusetts

*M. Michael Wolfe, MD (Chapter 4)*
Professor of Medicine
Case Western Reserve University
Chair, Department of Medicine
MetroHealth Medical Center
Cleveland, Ohio

# FOREWORD

The authors of *GI Emergencies: A Quick Reference Guide* have chosen a difficult task, namely to write a *vade mecum*. I am reminded of ancient times when a *vade mecum* would be used to help navigate a treacherous area. Well, the practice of medicine can be treacherous indeed in these litigious times, and a wrong decision can have fatal consequences not only for the patient but for the physician also. And so it becomes critical to have lodestones, guideposts, and *vade mecums*. This guidebook is of a size that can be easily tucked away, borne by the side pocket of a white jacket, but perhaps it will be transformed into an ebook for an ereader and accessed electronically. In either format, it is an easy read and guides the reader through all the emergencies a gastroenterologist commonly encounters. The student, house staff officer, and GI fellow will enjoy being guided by this book. No one should have to feel alone in times of important decision making.

Lawrence Brandt, MD
Professor of Medicine and Surgery
Albert Einstein College of Medicine
Bronx, New York

# INTRODUCTION

The handling of emergency situations is one of the most rewarding and challenging aspects of the practice of gastroenterology. Even experienced physicians feel a rush of adrenaline and a hint of nervousness when dealing with life-threatening illness, but this is magnified several-fold for the GI fellow early in his or her training. We have created this textbook to assist both the trainee and the experienced physician in the management of GI emergencies. Although many other textbooks have chapters dealing with the emergency conditions included in this book, we have chosen a unique format that is evidence-based yet practical and engaging. Each chapter is written by a GI fellow or resident along with a faculty member; we charged our trainee authors with emphasizing the elements of each topic that were the most important for a new fellow dealing with an emergent situation.

Each chapter begins with a clinical vignette in the form of a "call from the Emergency Department (ED)." After the case is presented, the text takes the reader through the initial approach to the problem (including what information you need from the ED and recommendations for diagnostic testing and management prior to seeing the patient). As the case unfolds, diagnostic and therapeutic recommendations are made, with a brief presentation of the best evidence that underlies our current practice. Last, we describe key "teaching points" that a GI specialist can use to educate house staff and other colleagues.

We believe that this unique format makes this book a guide to GI emergencies that is both practical and fun to read. The text can be read chapter-by-chapter, but it is also designed to be used "on-the-fly" when an emergency arises, guiding the GI specialist from the initial phone call to the final management decisions.

# 1

# Nonvariceal Upper Gastrointestinal Hemorrhage

*Pushpak Taunk, MD*
*Marcos C. Pedrosa, MD*

You receive the following call from the emergency department (ED):

> *We've got a 65-year-old woman with a past medical history of diabetes, hypertension, coronary artery disease (CAD), and rheumatoid arthritis who came in complaining of 3 days of black stools. Upon arriving to the ED, she also notes that today she has felt weak, light-headed, and dizzy. On exam, her blood pressure (BP) is 115/75, and her heart rate (HR) is 115.*

## INITIAL RESPONSE TO THE CALL

- Upper GI bleeding (UGIB) is associated with a mortality that is considered to be in the 5% to 10% range—proceed with urgency![1,2]

## WHAT INFORMATION DO YOU NEED IMMEDIATELY?

- HR and BP provide the most important information.[3]

Lowe RC, Farraye FA.
*GI Emergencies: A Quick Reference Guide* (pp 1-20).
© 2012 Taylor & Francis Group

- Determine the severity of blood loss: It is imperative to ask for vital signs with postural changes. If orthostatic (change in BP >10 mm Hg or HR >10 bpm from supine to standing), patient has lost at least 800 mL (15%) of circulating blood volume. Supine hypotension, tachycardia, tachypnea, and mental status changes suggest at least a 1500-mL (30%) loss of circulating blood volume.[4]
  - Recurrent bleeding can be predicted based on the severity of the initial bleeding episode. The patient's age, vital signs, and comorbidities are used to assess the severity of bleeding.[2]
  - Death from UGIB generally occurs because of decompensation of other illnesses. Exsanguination is rarely a cause of death in patients with UGIB.[3]
- Localization of source of bleeding: Distinguishes between upper and lower GI bleeding and guides further investigation.
  - Hematemesis: Bright red blood or coffee-ground emesis indicates that source of bleeding is likely proximal to the ligament of Treitz.[1] It confirms a UGI source of bleeding, assuming that the blood did not originate outside the GI tract (eg, nose bleed, hemoptysis, or upper respiratory tract source).[3]
  - Melena: Black, tarry, foul-smelling stools are often a manifestation of UGIB. As little as 50 to 100 mL of blood in the stomach can produce melena. Small bowel or proximal colonic source can also lead to stools that are difficult to differentiate from melena.[4] The presence of melena indicates that blood has been in the GI tract for at least 14 hours.[5]
  - Hematochezia: Bright red blood or maroon stools per rectum frequently indicate a lower GI source of bleeding. However, 10% to 15% of patients with hematochezia have a brisk UGI source of bleeding with hemodynamic instability.[4]
- Estimated duration of GI bleeding.[4]

# What Other Information Should Be Obtained for the Initial Evaluation?

- Symptoms of anemia: Fatigue, light-headedness, syncope, dyspnea, angina.[3]
- The presence or absence of abdominal or epigastric pain, gastroesophageal reflux disease (GERD)-related symptoms, persistent or severe vomiting.
- Other associated symptoms (ie, fever, weight loss).
- Medication use (eg, anticoagulants, anti-platelets, etc), including over-the-counter medications, such as nonsteroidal anti-inflammatory drugs (NSAIDs), aminosalicylic acid (ASA), and alcohol.[4]
- Relevant past medical history including prior GI bleeds, peptic ulcer disease (PUD), liver disease, recent procedures (eg, esophagogastroduodenoscopy [EGD], polypectomy, sphincterotomy), abdominal surgery (abdominal aortic aneurysms repair with graft), radiation therapy, inflammatory bowel disease.[4]
- Digital rectal examination for determination of stool color.[4]
- Initial laboratory result—complete blood count,** chemistry panel liver function tests, coagulation studies, type, and cross.

**The first hemoglobin (Hb)/hematocrit (Hct) measurement may be normal or minimally decreased because "people bleed whole blood," but it will decrease gradually to a stable level over 24 to 48 hours. As extravascular fluid enters the vascular space to restore volume, the Hb levels fall.[3,4]

# What Should You Tell the Team to Do Before You Get There?

- Ensure that the patient has 2 large-bore intravenous (IV) catheters (18 gauge or larger).[4]
- If patient is in shock, central venous access should be established.[4]
- Achieve adequate resuscitation with isotonic, crystalloid solutions and blood products (packed red blood cells).[4]

- Initial goal is resuscitation with resolution of hemodynamic instability to minimize complications.
- The need and degree of transfusion is not predicated solely upon the Hct level but is influenced by the bleeding acuity and rate, vital signs, and the presence of comorbidities, especially CAD.[6,7]
- Correct severe coagulopathy typically found in cirrhotic or anticoagulated patients with fresh frozen plasma.[4]
- Consider tracheal intubation to protect airway in patients with massive or variceal bleed, shock, and unstable or altered mental status.
- Consider nasogastric (NG) tube placement when the source of bleeding is uncertain.
  - Eighty percent are sensitive for active UGIB.[8]
  - NG aspirates that are grossly bloody or coffee grounds confirm a UGI source.[3]
  - However, the absence of blood does not by itself rule out the presence of a UGI source. Blood from a duodenal bulb ulcer may not flow back through the pylorus into the stomach.[4]
  - Up to 18% of UGIB have a nonbloody NG aspirate. Although some authors suggest that a nonbloody bile-stained aspirate rules out a duodenal source, physicians are incorrect about 50% of the time when they report bile in the aspirate.[9]
- Keep patient NPO (fasting), consider oxygen supplementation, Foley catheter.
- Stomach contents can be evacuated before EGD by use of NG tube saline lavage. If that fails, employ IV administration of erythromycin, used as a prokinetic agent, at a dose of 250 mg.[10,11]
- In general, chemical tests for occult blood in the stool guaiac or gastric aspirate (gastroccult) are NOT helpful. Both have high false-positive and false-negative rates, so always ask or check if there is gross blood, coffee grounds, melena, or hematochezia.[12]

- Proton pump inhibitor (PPI) therapy is recommended for all patients with UGIB.
- A recent study has shown that an IV PPI given before endoscopic therapy in patients with UGIB can reduce signs of bleeding ("downstage bleeding lesions") and the need for endoscopic therapy. However, there was no significant difference in transfusion requirements, rebleeding rate, surgery, or death.[13]
- IV PPI decreases the rebleeding and mortality following endoscopic therapy for high-risk lesions (stigmata of recent hemorrhage [SRH], high-risk stigmata).
- PPI dosing: Pantoprazole 80 mg bolus and 8 mg/hr infusion.
- If there is no rebleeding within 24 hours, the patient may be switched to oral pantoprazole 40 mg/day.

# DIAGNOSTIC AND THERAPEUTIC INTERVENTIONS

- Upper endoscopy is the primary diagnostic and therapeutic intervention.
  - Treatment aim is to stop ongoing bleeding.
  - Surgical referral if bleeding cannot be controlled.
  - Timing of endoscopy is controversial.[14]
    - No randomized controlled trials (RCTs) have confirmed that early endoscopy improves clinical outcomes.
    - However, there is a significant benefit of endoscopic therapy in high-risk patients that supports early endoscopy as beneficial in patients with high-risk clinical features (age >60, multiple comorbid illnesses, bleeding when hospitalized, severe coagulopathy, hypotension).

- Nevertheless, it is suggested that patients with clinical evidence of severe bleeding (tachycardia, hypotension, orthostatic changes) undergo an endoscopy soon after resuscitation and volume stabilization.[3]
- Ongoing bleeding, recurrent bleeding, bleeding in a patient hospitalized for other illness, severe comorbid illness, clinical suspicion of varices, and high clinical risk should also undergo urgent endoscopy.[8]
- Early endoscopy (admit and perform endoscopy within 24 hours) can be done in patients with low clinical risk, no severe comorbidities, and low volume bleed and in those who are hemodynamically stable or easily stabilized.[8]

  o Risks of endoscopy are increased in patients with UGIB due to the obscured field from blood and prolonged procedures and the need for prolonged sedation on an already frail patient.
  - Risks include aspiration; perforation and further bleeding from therapeutic intervention; and cardiovascular events, especially in patients with CAD.
  - Unstable patients benefit from anesthesia service consultation and sedation support.

  o Contraindications to endoscopy: Uncorrected coagulopathy (relative contraindication), unstable cardiac disease, or recent myocardial infarction (relative contraindication).[8]

- Angiography: Angiographic transcatheter embolization is a therapeutic option in patients who do not respond to endoscopic hemostasis and are otherwise poor candidates for surgery.[15]
- Capsule endoscopy and enteroscopy may be needed in patients with nonrevealing EGD and persistent UGIB.

## Sources of Nonvariceal Upper Gastrointestinal Bleeding

- Peptic ulcers are the most common etiology of UGIB, constituting approximately 40% to 55% of acute UGIB cases.[16,17]
- Mallory-Weiss tears: Longitudinal mucosal lacerations in the distal esophagus/proximal stomach associated with forceful retching typically seen in alcoholics and associated with hiatal hernias.
- Dieulafoy's lesion: A submucosal artery that erodes the overlying epithelium of the stomach; usually located in the gastric cardia within 7 cm of the gastroesophageal junction, but may occur anywhere in the GI tract.
- Aortoenteric fistula: Should be considered in all patients with a history of massive UGIB and a history of thoracic or abdominal aortic aneurysm, or prosthetic vascular graft.
- Hemorrhagic and erosive gastropathy: These lesions are restricted to the mucosa where no large blood vessels are present and, therefore, do not cause major bleeding[4] and are usually due to NSAIDs, alcohol, chemicals, or stress.[4]
- A complete listing of etiologies of UGIB is noted in Table 1-1.

## Why Do We Ultimately Choose Endoscopy?

- Although 80% to 90% of acute GI hemorrhage resolves spontaneously without recurrence, proper identification allows for risk stratification and allows for the identification of the patient at risk for further bleeding and endoscopic treatment in patients.[4]

**Table 1-1.**

# ETIOLOGIES OF UPPER GASTROINTESTINAL BLEEDING

| ESOPHAGEAL SOURCES | GASTRIC SOURCES | SMALL INTESTINAL SOURCES |
| --- | --- | --- |
| Peptic esophagitis with ulcers/erosion | Gastric ulcers (PUD):<br>- ASA/NSAIDs<br>- *Helicobacter pylori*<br>- Stress-induced ulcer<br>- Zollinger-Ellison syndrome | Duodenal ulcer |
| | | Angiodysplasia |
| | | Aortoenteric fistulas |
| | | Polyp or polypectomy |
| Pill induced:<br>- Alendronate<br>- Tetracycline<br>- Quinidine<br>- Potassium chloride<br>- Aspirin<br>- NSAIDs | Portal hypertension:<br>- Gastric varices<br>- Portal hypertensive gastropathy | Duodenal varices |
| | | Hemobilia |
| | | Hemosuccus pancreaticus |
| | | Malignancy |
| Infectious esophagitis:<br>- *Candida albicans*<br>- Herpes simplex<br>- HIV<br>- Cytomegalovirus | Vascular abnormalities:<br>- Angiodysplasia<br>- Dieulafoy's lesion<br>- Gastric antral vascular ectasia<br>- Osler-Weber-Rendu syndrome (HHT) | Bleeding from endoscopic biliary sphincterotomy |
| | | Blue rubber bleb nevus syndrome |
| Esophageal varices | Polyp and polypectomy | |
| Mallory-Weiss tear and Cameron lesions in hiatal hernia | Percutaneous endoscopic gastrostomy placement and pancreatic cyst drainage | |
| Malignancy | Malignancy | |

- PPI following endoscopic management for high-risk SRH decreases the risk for ulcer rebleeding, the need for urgent surgery, and the risk of death.[4]
- RCTs show that endoscopic therapy significantly improves outcomes, including further bleeding, transfusion, the need for surgery, the length of hospital stay, and costs in patients with high-risk bleeding ulcers (active bleeding, nonbleeding visible vessel, and possibly adherent clot).[18]

## PROGNOSTIC INFORMATION BASED ON ULCER APPEARANCE

- SRH are characteristics that provide information about the likelihood of a given lesion having caused the initial bleeding episode.[7]
- Various SRH and their bleeding risk are shown in Table 1-2.[19,20]
- SRH indicate the likelihood of continued bleeding or rebleeding.
- Approximately 33% of patients found to have an ulcer with active bleeding or a nonbleeding visible vessel will have further bleeding that requires surgery if treated expectantly.[21]
- Patients with clean-based ulcers very rarely rebleed, with rates close to zero.[3]

## DECIDING WHICH LESIONS ARE APPROPRIATE FOR THERAPEUTIC ENDOSCOPIC INTERVENTION

- Owing to a high risk of rebleeding, major SRH (active bleeding and nonbleeding visible vessel) mandate endoscopic therapy at the time of diagnosis.[22]

**Table 1-2.**

## STIGMATA OF RECENT HEMORRHAGE AND RISK OF BLEEDING IN PATIENTS WITH PEPTIC ULCERS

| ENDOSCOPIC SRH | RISK OF REBLEEDING OR CONTINUED BLEEDING AFTER ONLY MEDICAL THERAPY |
| --- | --- |
| **Major SRH** | |
| Active bleeding | 80% to 90% |
| Nonbleeding visible vessel | 40% to 60% |
| **Intermediate SRH** | |
| Adherent clot | 26% |
| Oozing of blood | 10% to 28% |
| **Minor SRH** | |
| Flat pigmented spot | 13% |
| **No SRH** | |
| Clean-based ulcer | 4% to 5% |

- Owing to a low risk of rebleeding, endoscopic therapy should NOT be performed for minor stigmata or recent hemorrhage (flat pigmented spot and clean-based ulcer).[22]
- The treatment of an adherent clot is controversial. Most endoscopists favor aggressive endoscopic clot removal.[23]
  - Why? Removal of adherent clot may reveal an unexpected high-risk lesion that has a high rebleeding rate and requires endoscopic treatment.[7]

# TECHNIQUES OF
# THERAPEUTIC ENDOSCOPY

- Techniques include injection therapy, ablative therapy, and mechanical (tamponade) therapy.
  - Injection therapy
    - Epinephrine is the most commonly used injection therapy.[7]
    - The agent promotes hemostasis by local tamponade secondary to vasospasm.
    - Epinephrine is generally used in a concentration of 1:10,000.
    - With systemic circulation, epinephrine can produce angina in patients with CAD, both by coronary vasospasm and by increasing myocardial workload. Other toxic effects include tachycardia, cardiac arrhythmias, and hypertension. This can be prevented with use of 12 mL or less of epinephrine.[24]
    - Epinephrine is reasonably effective in stopping the acute bleed, but bleeding may recur after injection as its local effect wears off (usually 20 minutes).[25,26]
    - Epinephrine injection alone does NOT provide optimal efficacy and should be used in combination with another modality.[27]
    - Endoscopists generally apply a second hemostatic technique to provide a more durable therapy.[7]
    - Other injection agents: Sclerosants, thrombin, fibrin glue, cyanoacrylate.
      - Sclerosants: Less effective than epinephrine and considered only in patients with severe CAD.[28]
  - Ablative therapy
    - Delivers intense energy to a bleeding site, which promotes hemostasis by coagulating

- tissue proteins, causing edema and vaso-constriction, activating thrombocoagulation, and destroying tissue.[29]
- Contact methods, including thermocoagulation and bipolar electrocoagulation (BICAP), require the probe to touch the tissue to deliver ablative energy.
- BICAP devices contain 2 electrodes on the probe tip. Electricity essentially travels from one electrode to the other, thereby minimizing stray electrical currents and scatter injury.
- The probe is placed directly on the ulcer at the site of major SRH. Endoscopists apply firm pressure during contact ablation to compress and weld the 2 sides of a bleeding vessel.
- Effective hemostasis is suggested by whitening of the lesion and flattening of a non-bleeding visible vessel or clot remnant.
- Trials have shown that both methods result in much higher rates of hemostasis than medical therapy.
- Argon plasma coagulation (APC) is used for elective treatment of angiodysplastic lesions or gastric vascular ectasia (watermelon stomach).[30]
  - o Mechanical therapy
    - A device mechanically compresses the bleeding source in a similar way to a tourniquet or suture.
    - Endoscopic clips (metallic hemoclips or endoclips) are currently the preferred mechanical therapy.[31,32]
      - □ Proper endoscopic clip placement requires a highly skilled endoscopist for placement at the correct angle and precise spot.[7]

- Endoscopic clips work like surgical clips in that they approximate 2 sides of a vessel to immediately and securely occlude bleeding.
- Endoscopic clips are best deployed enface rather than tangentially.
- The endoscopic clip should be opened and fully extended directly around the bleeding lesion so that the jaws are across the target and can be embedded into adjacent intact tissue.
- Beneficial endoscopic clip properties include rotatability, interlocking jaws for improved mechanical clamping, and reversibility (the device can be redeployed if it is initially improperly placed).[32]
- At least 2 endoscopic clips are placed to clamp an actively bleeding artery in an ulcer.

- Endoscopic clips are less successful for the treatment of fibrotic lesions, such as chronic ulcers, than for the treatment of inflammatory lesions, such as acute ulcers.[31]
- Endoscopic clips can dislodge within 1 day of application, and this drawback limits their efficacy.[33]
- The placement of these clips rarely produces complications other than failed therapy.[34]
- Elderly patients have an increased risk of endoscopic clip failure attributed to attenuated tissue integrity.[35]
- Endoscopic clips also mark lesions to direct angiographic or surgical therapy as they are radiographically opaque.[35]
- Endoscopic clips seem to be comparable in efficacy to thermocoagulation or electrocoagulation as monotherapy for patients with major SRH.[36]

- RCTs also indicate that, even after endoscopic therapy, a bolus of an IV PPI followed by a constant infusion of PPI for 72 hours will significantly lessen recurrent bleeding, but not mortality.[12]
- The hypothesis behind the use of high-dose constant infusion PPI therapy is based on older experimental studies that suggest that maintaining intragastric pH >6 will enhance clot formation and clot stability.[37]
- Routine second-look endoscopy is not recommended (Figure 1-1).[27]

## OTHER IMPORTANT INTERVENTIONS

- Prevention of recurrent bleeding in the long-term should focus on factors that cause ulcers: *H. pylori*, NSAIDs, and acid.
- Patients with bleeding peptic ulcers should be tested for *H. pylori* and should receive eradication if present, with subsequent confirmation of eradication.
- Patients with bleeding ulcers unrelated to *H. pylori* or NSAIDs should remain on full-dose antisecretory therapy indefinitely.

## POSTDISCHARGE RECOMMENDATIONS

- In patients with previous ulcer bleeding who require an NSAID, it should be recognized that treatment with a traditional NSAID plus PPI or a cyclooxygenase 2 (COX-2) inhibitor alone is still associated with a clinically important risk for recurrent ulcer bleeding.
- In patients with previous ulcer bleeding who require an NSAID, the combination of a PPI and a COX-2 inhibitor is recommended to reduce the risk for recurrent bleeding from that of COX-2 inhibitors alone.

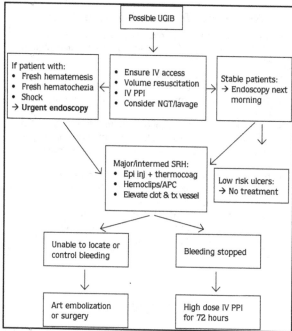

**Figure 1-1.** Approach to nonvariceal GI bleeding. (Adapted from Sung JJY. How I do it: management of upper gastrointestinal bleeding. http://www.worldendo.org/assets/downloads/pdf/publications/how_i_doit/2008/omed_hid_upper%20gastrointestinal_bleeding.pdf. Accessed May 19, 2011.)

- In patients who receive low-dose ASA and develop acute ulcer bleeding, ASA therapy should be restarted as soon as the risk for cardiovascular complication is thought to outweigh the risk for bleeding.[27]
- In patients with previous ulcer bleeding who require cardiovascular prophylaxis, it should be recognized that clopidogrel alone has a higher risk for rebleeding than ASA combined with a PPI.

---

### *Key Points for the Referring Team*

- It is important to determine the severity of blood loss in patients based on vital signs, orthostatics, and mental status.
- Aggressive hemodynamic stabilization through 2 large bore IVs is imperative prior to endoscopic intervention.
- The initial Hb/Hct may not reflect the degree of blood loss.
- Hematemesis, melena, and hematochezia may aid in identifying the location of bleeding, although both upper and lower GI bleeding can present with melena and hematochezia.
- Placement of a NG tube is generally not very helpful in determining the source of bleeding, but may aid when the diagnosis is uncertain.
- IV PPIs are important for the prevention of recurrent bleeding; however, they do not affect mortality.
- Use a team approach—especially for complicated patients.

---

# REFERENCES

1. Longstreth GF. Epidemiology of hospitalizations for acute upper gastrointestinal hemorrhage: a population-based study. *Am J Gastroenterol.* 1995;90:206-210.
2. Rockall TA, Logan RF, Devlin HB, et al. Risk assessment after acute upper gastrointestinal hemorrhage. *Gut.* 1996;38:316-321.
3. Laine L. Upper gastrointestinal bleeding. *ASGE: Clinical Update.* 2007;14:1-4.
4. Moore TC, Tseng C, Wolfe MM. Gastrointestinal hemorrhage. *Cecil's Essentials.* 2010;34:385-388.
5. Hilsman, JH. The color of blood-containing feces following the instillation of citrated blood at various levels of the small intestine. *Gastroenterology.* 1950;15:131-134.
6. Hogue CW, Goodnough LT, Monk TG. Preoperative myocardial ischemic episodes are related to hematocrit levels in patients undergoing radical prostatectomy. *Transfusion.* 1998;38:924-931.
7. Cappell MS. Therapeutic endoscopy for acute upper gastrointestinal bleeding. *Nature Reviews: Gastroenterology & Hepatology.* 2010;7:214-229.

8.  Van Dam J. Endoscopic therapy for non-variceal acute upper GI bleeding. In: Van Dam J, Wong RCK, eds. *Gastrointestinal Endoscopy*. Austin, TX: Landes Bioscience; 2004:75-81.

9.  Cuellar RE, Gavaler JS, Alexander JA, et al. Gastrointestinal tract hemorrhage. The value of a nasogastric aspirate. *Arch Intern Med*. 1990;150:1381-1384.

10. Coffin B, Pocard M, Panis Y, et al. Erythromycin improves the quality of EGD in patients with acute upper GI bleeding: a randomized controlled study. *Gastrointest Endosc*. 2002;56:174-179.

11. Winstead NS, Wilcox CM. Erythromycin prior to endoscopy for acute gastrointestinal hemorrhage: a cost effective analysis. *Aliment Pharmacol Ther*. 2007;26:1371-1377.

12. Lau JYW, Sung JJ, Lee KK, et al. Effect of intravenous omeprazole on recurrent bleeding after endoscopic treatment of bleeding peptic ulcers. *N Engl J Med*. 2000;343:310-316.

13. Lau JY, Leung WK, Wu JC, et al. Omeprazole before endoscopy in patients with gastrointestinal bleeding. *N Engl J Med*. 2007;356:1631-1640.

14. Spiegel BM, Vakil NB, Ofman JJ. Endoscopy for acute nonvariceal upper gastrointestinal hemorrhage: is sooner better? A systematic review. *Arch Intern Med*. 2001;161:1393-1404.

15. Sung JJY. How I do it: management of upper gastrointestinal bleeding. http://www.worldendo.org/assets/downloads/pdf/publications/how_i_doit/2008/omed_hid_upper%20gastrointestinal_bleeding.pdf. Accessed May 19, 2011.

16. Enestvedt BK, Grainek IM, Mattek N, et al. An evaluation of endoscopic indications and findings related to nonvariceal upper GI hemorrhage in a large multicenter consortium. *Gastrointest Endosc*. 2008;67:422-429.

17. Jutabha R, Jensen DM. Management of upper gastrointestinal bleeding in the patient with chronic liver disease. *Med Clin North Am*. 1996;80:1035-1068.

18. Cook DJ, Salena B, Guyatt GH, et al. Endoscopic therapy for acute non-variceal upper gastrointestinal hemorrhage: a meta-analysis. *Gastroenterology*. 1992;102:139-148.

19. Kovacs TO, Jensen DM. Endoscopic treatment of ulcer bleeding. *Curr Treat Options Gastroenterol*. 2007;10:143-148.

20. Leontiadis GI, Howden CW. Pharmacologic treatment of peptic ulcer bleeding. *Curr Treat Options Gastroenterol*. 2007;10:134-142.

21. Laine L, Peterson W. Bleeding peptic ulcers. *N Engl J Med*. 1994;331:717-727.

22. Freeman ML. Stigmata of hemorrhage in bleeding ulcers. *Gastrointest Endosc Clin North Am.* 1997;7:559-574.

23. Kahi CJ, Jensen DM, Sung JJ, et al. Endoscopic therapy versus medical therapy for bleeding peptic ulcer with adherent clot: a meta-analysis. *Gastroenterology.* 2005;129:855-862.

24. Cappell MS, Lacovone FM. Safety and efficacy of esophago-gastroduodenoscopy after myocardial infarction. *Am J Med.* 1999;106:29-35.

25. Calvet X, Vergara M, Brullet E, et al. Addition of a second endoscopic treatment following epinephrine injection improves outcome in high-risk bleeding ulcers. *Gastroenterology.* 2004;126:441-450.

26. Cappell MS, Friedel D. Acute nonvariceal upper gastrointestinal bleeding: endoscopic diagnosis and therapy. *Med Clin North Am.* 2008;92:511-550.

27. Barkun A, Bardou M, Kuipers E, et al. International consensus on the management of patients with nonvariceal upper gastrointestinal bleeding. *Ann Intern Med.* 2010;152:101-113.

28. Lious TC, Chang WH, Want HY, et al. Large-volume endoscopic injection of epinephrine plus normal saline for peptic ulcer bleeding. *J Gastroenterol Hepatol.* 2007;22:996-1002.

29. Jensen DM, Machicado GA. Endoscopic hemostasis of ulcer hemorrhage with injection, thermal and combination methods. *Tech Gastrointest Endosc.* 2005;7:124-131.

30. Kwan V, Bourke MJ, Williams SJ, et al. Argon plasma coagulation in the management of symptomatic gastrointestinal vascular lesions: experience in 100 consecutive patients with long-term follow-up. *Am J Gastroenterol.* 2006;101:58-63.

31. Jensen DM, Machicado GA, Hirabayashi K. Hemoclipping (CLIP) of chronic ulcers: a randomized prospective study of initial success, CLIP retention rates, and ulcer healing. *Gastrointest Endosc.* 2005;61:174.

32. Conway JD, Adler DG, Diehl DL, et al. Technology status evaluation report: endoscopic hemostatic devices. *Gastrointest Endosc.* 2009;69(6):987-996.

33. Chen CY, Yau KK, Siu WT, et al. Endoscopic hemostasis by using the TriClip for peptic ulcer hemorrhage: a pilot study. *Gastrointest Endosc.* 2008;67:35-39.

34. Ishiguro T, Nagawa H. Inadvertent endoscopic application of a hemoclip to the splenic artery through a perforated gastric ulcer. *Gastrointest Endosc.* 2001;53:378-379.

35. Eriksson LG, Sundborn M, Gustavsson S, et al. Endoscopic marking with a metallic clip facilitates transcatheter arterial embolization in upper peptic ulcer bleeding. *J Vasc Interven Radiol.* 2006;17:959-964.
36. Lin HJ, Hsieh YH, Tseng GY, Perng CL, Chang FY, Lee SD. A prospective randomized trial of endoscopic hemoclip versus heater probe thermocoagulation for peptic ulcer bleeding. *Am J Gastroenterol.* 2002;97:2250-2254.
37. Green FW, Kaplan MM, Curtis LE, et al. Effect of acid and pepsin on blood coagulation and platelet aggregation. A possible contributor prolonged gastroduodenal mucosal hemorrhage. *Gastroenterology.* 1978;74:38-43.

# 2

# Evaluation and Management of Acute Variceal Hemorrhage

*Ashraf Saleemuddin, MD*
*Uri Avissar, MD*

You receive the following call from the emergency department (ED):

*A 57-year-old woman with primary biliary cirrhosis (PBC) presents with malaise and dizziness following an episode of hematemesis earlier in the day.*

*She was diagnosed with PBC 9 years ago after evaluation for fatigue and an elevated alkaline phosphatase level. At the time, a liver biopsy demonstrated cirrhosis. She currently has adequate liver synthetic function and shows no evidence of liver decompensation. Her last endoscopy was about 2 years prior and was notable for small esophageal varices.*

*Today, she felt nauseated an hour after eating dinner and vomited about 1 cup of bright red blood. She then began to feel very dizzy and light-headed and was driven to the ED by her husband. In triage, she passed a large amount of melena.*

Lowe RC, Farraye FA.
*GI Emergencies: A Quick Reference Guide* (pp 21-46).
© 2012 Taylor & Francis Group

*She denies any recent nonsteroidal anti-inflammatory drug (NSAID) use, fever, chills, chest pain, or shortness of breath.*

*Physical Exam:*

*VS: T 97.5; HR 105; BP 86/43; RR 20; O$_2$Sat 96%/RA*

*GENERAL: frail, lethargic-appearing woman lying in bed*

*HEENT: sclera icteric*

*COR: nl S1S2, RRR, no murmurs*

*LUNG: clear to auscultation*

*ABD: normoactive BS, nontender, mild distension, no hepatosplenomegaly*

*EXTREM: no edema*

*SKIN: jaundiced*

*RECTAL: no masses, melenic stool in vault*

*NEURO: no asterixis*

*Her hemoglobin was 9.1 and her hematocrit was 26.0 with a normal white blood cell count and platelets. The chemistries were normal. The liver enzyme panel was remarkable for AST 49, ALT 32, alkaline phosphatase 371, total bilirubin 2.2 (direct 1.8), albumin 3.7, and INR 1.16.*

The above case requires your timely medical management in several different capacities, including the emergent intervention to stabilize a critically ill patient, the appropriate workup and diagnosis in the setting of hematemesis, the initiation of remedial therapies or procedures, and the implementation of prophylactic measures to prevent future complications or recurrence. However, before we can effectively treat this patient, we must have a firm understanding of the underlying condition.

## NATURAL HISTORY OF VARICES

An acute upper gastrointestinal bleed (UGIB) in the setting of portal hypertension or cirrhosis raises the concern for an acute variceal hemorrhage. Liver cirrhosis is the leading cause of portal hypertension, although there are many other possible etiologies. Portal hypertension results from physiologic changes causing an increase in both portal vascular resistance and portal blood flow. Increases in portal vascular resistance can be attributed to structural factors, such as liver fibrosis and regenerative nodule formation, as well as dynamic factors, including endothelial dysfunction leading to elevated hepatic vascular tone. Concomitantly, portal blood flow increases drastically due to splanchnic vasodilatation and increased cardiac output. Ultimately, these physiologic changes lead to the formation of gastroesophageal varices (GOV), which serve as collaterals between the portal and systemic venous systems and help alleviate the volume and pressure overload on the portal vasculature. Nevertheless, as portal pressure increases, these varices grow in size and their vessel wall thins. This results in increased wall tension and eventual rupture.

Portal hypertension can be measured by determining the hepatic venous pressure gradient (HVPG), though the procedure is invasive. HVPG is calculated with a balloon catheter by measuring both the free hepatic vein pressure (FHVP) and the wedged hepatic venous pressure (WHVP) as follows:

$$HVPG = WHVP - FHVP$$

- Portal hypertension is defined by a HVPG greater than 5 mm Hg. A HVPG greater than 10 mm Hg predisposes to the development of varices, while a HVPG greater than 20 mm Hg is a poor prognostic factor during a variceal bleed.[1]

  The prevalence of varices and the incidence of variceal bleeds in the setting of liver cirrhosis are summarized in Figure 2-1.

- The prevalence of varices is higher among patients with advanced stages of cirrhosis as defined by the Child-Pugh classification, which considers the grade of encephalopathy, presence of ascites, serum bilirubin and albumin levels, and INR.

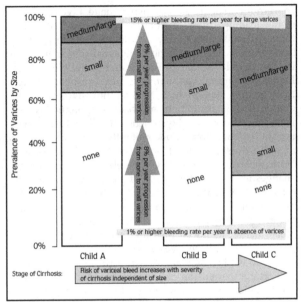

**Figure 2-1.** Prevalence of varices by size and stage of cirrhosis. Rate of progression of varices and rate of bleeding is also shown. (Adapted from Patrick S. Kamath lecture notes on Portal Hypertension Bleeding at the Transplant Hepatology Certification Review Course, September 2008.)

- Nearly half of all patients with liver cirrhosis have varices at the time of diagnosis, and data show that varices develop at a rate of 8% per year and progress from small to large varices at the same rate.[2]
- The incidence of variceal bleeding ranges from 5% to 15% per year in cirrhotic patients and is influenced primarily by the size of varices, though the stage of cirrhosis and presence of red wale marks on endoscopy are independent risk factors.[3]

- Although variceal hemorrhage may stop spontaneously in up to 40% of patients, rebleeding occurs in
  up to 60% of untreated patients within the following
  year. The risk of rebleeding is highest within the
  first 2 weeks after the initial episode of bleeding.
  Despite therapeutic advances, mortality at 6 weeks
  after the index bleed is approximately 20%.

*Assuming this patient is indeed suffering from an
esophageal variceal bleed, you may wonder if preventative measures against variceal bleeds could
have been implemented in this case. We will return
to this matter later in the chapter, but first we must
focus our attention on providing emergent care for
this critically ill patient. Remember, her 6-week
mortality rate is nearly 20%, so what is your plan?*

# MANAGEMENT OF
# ACUTE VARICEAL BLEEDS

Goals of therapy:
- Volume resuscitation
- Control bleeding
- Prevent early rebleeding
- Prevent complications associated with bleeding.

Figure 2-2 provides an algorithm to help guide the
management of acute variceal bleed.

## RESUSCITATION

- Patients with significant GI bleeds are best managed with at least 2 venous access sites, preferably
  with large-bore peripheral intravenous (IV) access
  catheters.
- The initial laboratory assessment should include a
  complete blood count (CBC), complete metabolic
  panel (CMP; including renal and liver function
  tests), and coagulation panel.

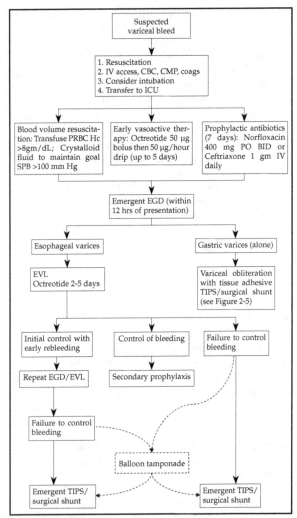

**Figure 2-2.** Management of acute variceal bleeding.

- Crystalloid fluids should be initially administered to maintain a systolic blood pressure of 100 mm Hg and a heart rate below 110 bpm.
  - Over-resuscitation with crystalloid fluids and blood products may lead to an elevated portal pressure and precipitate recurrent variceal hemorrhage or exacerbate ascites and extravascular edema.[3]
- Blood transfusions should be administered to maintain hemodynamic stability and hemoglobin levels of approximately 8 g/dL.
  - Again, a conservative goal of 8 g/dL helps avoid increases in portal pressure with a potential to exacerbate variceal bleeding or cause extravascular fluid overload.
- We would suggest having a low threshold for elective endotracheal intubation in order to protect the airway, as the risk of aspiration is high in the presence of encephalopathy, hematemesis, and during an emergent endoscopy.
- The transfusion of fresh frozen plasma should be considered in patients with significant coagulopathy.
- Platelet transfusion may be considered in patients with a low platelet count (<50,000).
- Studies have not shown a beneficial effect of recombinant activated factor VII (rFVIIa).[4]
- ICU admission is warranted when a variceal bleed is suspected.

*While stabilizing the patient with resuscitative measures, steps to control the bleeding are implemented concomitantly. Although endoscopy is the definitive therapy, pharmacologic advances have led to a repertoire of drugs at your disposal, which should be administered immediately when you suspect variceal bleeding.*

## Pharmacologic Therapy

- The goal of pharmacologic therapy is to reduce portal blood flow by inducing splanchnic vasoconstriction.
- Octreotide, a somatostatin analogue, has splanchnic vasoconstrictive effects and is the only drug of its class available for use in the United States.
  - Octreotide is administered with a loading dose IV bolus of 50 µg followed by a continuous infusion of 50 µg/hour (see Table 2-1 for further details).
  - Octreotide is well-tolerated and can be used for up to 5 days with a limited side effect profile.[5]
  - Octreotide is associated with rapid tachyphylaxis, and its vasoactive effects are likely transient, lasting less than 5 minutes.[6]
  - Nevertheless, octreotide use in combination with urgent endoscopy has been shown to improve hemostasis and reduce the rate of early rebleeding compared to endoscopy alone. However, the rates of mortality and other adverse events remain unchanged.[7]
- Other vasoconstrictors used with or without nitrates, such as vasopressin, are limited by multiple side effects and severe complications. These complications include cardiac arrhythmias as well as myocardial, internal organ, and peripheral ischemia. Terlipressin, a vasopressin analogue with a longer half-life, has a milder side effect profile but is not currently available for use in the United States.
- Under no circumstance should β-blockers be administered during an acute variceal bleed because they will oppose the appropriate physiological response to hypovolemic shock in the setting of bleeding. β-blockers can be started or resumed only after discontinuation of the octreotide drip or shortly before the patient is discharged.

Table 2-1.

## GASTROENTEROLOGIST'S TOOLBOX FOR ACUTE VARICEAL BLEED

| AGENT | DOSE | DURATION | SIDE EFFECTS/COMPLICATIONS | COMMENTS |
|-------|------|----------|----------------------------|----------|
| **Primary and Secondary Prophylaxis Agents** | | | | |
| Propranolol | 20 mg given orally twice a day increased to maximum tolerated until HR 55 to 65 bpm | Indefinite | • Bradycardia, hypotension, and heart failure<br>• Fatigue and depression as side effects are more common in cirrhotic patients | Monitor HR with titration |
| Nadolol | 40 mg given orally once a day increased to maximum tolerated until HR 55 to 65 bpm | Indefinite | • Bronchospasm may exacerbate pulmonary disease<br>• In diabetes, may lead to or mask symptoms of hypoglycemia | Monitor HR with titration |
| Isosorbide mononitrate | 10 mg given orally every night increased to a maximum of 20 mg twice a day | Indefinite | • Sexual dysfunction and impotence | To be used in association with ß-blocker |
| Endoscopic variceal ligation | Every 2 to 4 weeks; first surveillance EGD 1 to 3 months after obliteration, then every 6 to 12 months | Until variceal obliteration | Esophageal perforation, ulceration, mild transient dysphagia, and chest discomfort | After procedure, start liquids and advance to regular diet within a day |

(continued)

Table 2-1. *(continued)*

## Gastroenterologist's Toolbox for Acute Variceal Bleed

| AGENT | DOSE | DURATION | SIDE EFFECTS/COMPLICATIONS | COMMENTS |
|---|---|---|---|---|
| **Vasoactive Agents** | | | | |
| Octreotide | 50 µg IV bolus followed by infusion of 50 µg/hr | 2 to 5 days | Cardiac arrhythmias, hyperglycemia, GI distress (nausea, diarrhea, abdominal cramping). | Available in the United States |
| Somatostatin | 250 mg IV bolus followed by infusion of 250 mg/hr | 2 to 5 days | headache, pruritus | Not available in the United States |
| Terlipressin | 2 mg IV every 4 hrs for 48 hrs, followed by 1 mg IV every 4 hrs | 2 to 5 days | Cardiac arrhythmias, myocardial ischemia, headache, GI distress (diarrhea, abdominal cramping) | Not available in the United States |
| **Prophylactic Antibiotics** | | | | |
| Norfloxacin | 400 mg given orally twice a day | 7 days | Headache, dizziness, GI distress (nausea, abdominal cramping). transaminitis | Used in patients with low probability of quinolone resistance |
| Ceftriaxone | 1 g IV once a day | 7 days | Rash, diarrhea, transaminitis, eosinophilia | Used in patients with high probability of quinolone resistance |

# ENDOSCOPIC THERAPY

- Endoscopic evaluation should occur as soon as possible within the first 12 hours of a patient presenting with an acute variceal bleed.
- Endoscopic treatments are successful in controlling bleeding in 80% to 90% of cases.[8]
- Endoscopic variceal ligation (EVL) is the current standard of care.
  - Varices are banded using a multi-shot device starting at the level of the gastroesophageal (GE) junction and moving upward in the esophagus.
  - Bands should be placed as proximally as possible, and all 4 quadrants should be treated circumferentially around the esophagus.
  - In general, banding sites should be at least 2 cm apart to include an adequate amount of mucosa in the band.
  - The bands occlude variceal blood flow and lead to ischemia and necrosis of the mucosa and submucosa. Both the elastic bands and necrotic tissue slough off over a period of 2 to 3 weeks, leaving shallow ulcerations called esophageal band ulcers.
  - Chest discomfort or mild dysphagia is common in the first few days following the procedure.
  - Bleeding can occur at the site of band ulcers but is typically less severe than the index variceal bleed.
  - EVL is repeated in 1 to 2 weeks and every 2 weeks thereafter to re-evaluate and obliterate the varices.
- Studies suggest that EVL is more effective than endoscopic injection sclerotherapy in controlling bleeding. Sclerotherapy is also associated with slightly higher rates of complications compared to EVL, such as esophageal ulcer bleeding.[9] One advantage of sclerotherapy is a wider field of vision than the

banding device. When a variceal bleed is difficult to control or localize with EVL, it is reasonable to try sclerotherapy during a second attempt at endoscopic treatment.

- We are often asked about placement of a nasoduodenal feeding tube or nasogastric (NG) tube after EVL. Recent EVL is not a contraindication for nasoduodenal or NG tube placement, and it can be placed if necessary.

*Endoscopy confirmed bleeding esophageal varices. We performed EVL on our patient, and the placement of 6 bands stopped the bleeding. Now, we must focus our attention on reducing the risk of future complications and recurrence. First and foremost, we must consider antibiotics.*

## ANTIBIOTIC PROPHYLAXIS

- Bacterial infections are a common and severe complication among cirrhotic patients presenting with a UGIB irrespective of cause (variceal or nonvariceal).
  - o Approximately one-fifth of cirrhotic patients with UGIB have a bacterial infection upon presentation, and nearly half acquire nosocomial infections during hospitalization.[9]
  - o Endoscopy further increases the risk of infection.
  - o The most prevalent infections include urinary tract infections, spontaneous bacterial peritonitis, aspiration pneumonia, and bacteremia.
- Bacterial infections in this setting of variceal bleeds greatly increase the rate of recurrence and mortality. Patients with a Child-Pugh class of B or C carry the highest risk of rebleeding.
- Short-term antibiotics should always be administered to cirrhotic patients with a UGIB whether ascites is present or not.

- Norfloxacin is a reasonable choice of antibiotic and can be administered at a dose of 400 mg orally twice daily for 7 days. Other options of IV and oral antibiotics are listed in Table 2-1.
- In high-risk patients, IV ceftriaxone at 1 g/day may be a better choice.[3]

*We treated our patient with antibiotics, and there has been no further bleeding during the following day. But what if we were not able to control the bleeding during the initial endoscopy? After additional attempts of EVL or sclerotherapy, what if she had recurrent episodes of bleeding? What else can we do for our patient?*

## SALVAGE THERAPIES

### *Transjugular Intrahepatic Portosystemic Shunt*

- Transjugular intrahepatic portosystemic shunt (TIPS) is the preferred rescue therapy upon failure to control bleeding or rebleeding by standard management with endoscopic and pharmacologic interventions.
- Mortality rates after TIPS remain high at 30% to 50%, although this measure is likely inflated due to the selection bias inherent in this severely ill patient cohort.
- Cirrhotic patients in Child-Pugh class B or C with persistent bleeding after endoscopy are at the highest risk for treatment failure. Early intervention with TIPS may improve outcome and mortality.[10] However, in Child-Pugh C cirrhotic patients, outcomes remain very poor, and TIPS is plagued with complications. We generally do not use TIPS in this group unless it serves as a bridge therapy to a forthcoming liver transplant.
- TIPS is contraindicated in the presence of hepatopulmonary syndrome or pulmonary hypertension. Presence or history of hepatic encephalopathy should also dissuade from its use. TIPS placement

**Table 2-2.**

## CONTRAINDICATION FOR TRANSJUGULAR INTRAHEPATIC PORTOSYSTEMIC SHUNT

| TIPS CONTRAINDICATIONS |
| --- |
| Cardiopulmonary disease |
|     Advanced heart failure |
|     Severe pulmonary hypertension |
|     Hepatopulmonary syndrome |
| Hepatic vascular compromise |
|     Hepatic artery or celiac axis occlusion/thrombosis |
| Current or previous hepatic encephalopathy |
| Advanced cirrhosis (Child-Pugh class C) |
| Active systemic infection |
|     Hepatic abscess |
| Pre-hepatic portal hypertension |
| Polycystic liver disease |
| *RELATIVE CONTRAINDICATIONS* |
| Hepatocellular carcinoma |
| Age >65 |
| Total bilirubin >3 mg/dL |

should be postponed in the setting of active infection until the infection is properly treated. A more comprehensive list of contraindications for TIPS is shown in Table 2-2.

*When faced with uncontrolled bleeding despite your best efforts, a member of the critical care team may ask you about balloon tamponade. Balloon tamponade should be considered only after all pharmacologic and endoscopic interventions have been exhausted. Balloon tamponade will only buy you a few more hours. If you believe you can attain a more definitive treatment, such as TIPS, and control bleeding within those hours, then consider tamponade. Balloon tamponade may be an important transient measure in patients whom you believe the short- and long-term outcome is likely to be good once bleeding is controlled. Good candidates are those without other comorbidities or complications or a transplant candidate. This, however, is by far the exception. In most cases, balloon tamponade is a futile measure. It frequently leads to fatal complications and should only be performed by an experienced practitioner.*

### Balloon Tamponade

- Balloon tamponade is a transient measure used exclusively in the setting of uncontrolled bleeding and failed standard therapy when definitive treatment, such as TIPS, is anticipated within a day.
- Remember, you can only use it for about 12 hours.
- The patient should be intubated before placement of balloon tamponade.
- The Minnesota tube is different from the Sengstaken-Blakemore tube in that it has 4 lumens with an additional esophageal aspiration port.
- A brief review of Minnesota tube placement is shown in Figure 2-3.[11]
- Esophageal balloon inflation can cause major complications, including esophageal rupture and necrosis.

*As we previously noted, there are preventative measures against variceal bleeding that should have been initiated with our patient. The risk of variceal bleeding in patients with liver cirrhosis is well-established. Given her history of PBC, how should she have been managed prior to her episode of hematemesis?*

**A**
1. Preparation before insertion:
   a. Test balloons under water for leaks.
   b. Insufflate gastric balloon sump syringe to 100 cc through the large bore gastric balloon port (3a) and clamp port. With a monometer attached to the narrow bore gastric balloon port (3b), measure the pressure. Continue insufflating to 400 cc while measuring pressure at 100 cc intervals. Deflate gastric balloon.
2. Insertion
   a. Insert tube via mouth into the stomach as far as 50 cm mark or further.
   b. Insufflate the gastric balloon through the wide port while the manometer is attached to the narrow port to 100 cc. Confirm that pressure is not more than 15 mm Hg higher than measured before insertion at the same volume (100 cc).
   c. Continue insufflating to 450 cc while checking pressure at 100 cc intervals to make sure it does not exceed the correlating measurements before insertion by 15 mm Hg. Clamp ports.
3. Placement
   a. Pull tube to create enough tension so that the gastric balloon is pressing on the gastric cardia tightly.
   b. Secure tube with cloth tape to a foam pad or football helmet.
   c. Confirm position of gastric balloon with chest and abdominal x-ray.
4. Esophageal balloon
   a. If bleeding is not controlled, esophageal balloon tamponade can be attempted.
   b. Insufflate the esophageal balloon through the wide port (4a) while the manometer is attached to the narrow port (4b) to a pressure of 25 to 35 mm Hg and clamp ports.
5. Balloon tamponade care
   a. Esophageal balloon tamponade should not be continued for more than 12 hours.
   b. Esophageal balloon should be deflated every 2 hours for 10 minutes, then re-inflated as above.
   c. X-rays should be repeated every 4 hours for monitoring.

**B**

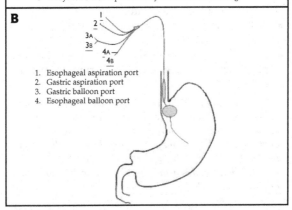

1. Esophageal aspiration port
2. Gastric aspiration port
3. Gastric balloon port
4. Esophageal balloon port

**Figure 2-3.** Minnesota tube placement. (Adapted from University of South Alabama Gastroenterology Continuing Education Site.)

# PRIMARY PROPHYLAXIS

- Once a patient is diagnosed with cirrhosis, screening for varices with endoscopy is performed to check for the presence and grade of varices. Figure 2-4 details the current screening and prophylactic recommendations for varices.
    - The stage of cirrhosis guides the frequency of screening endoscopy after the initial diagnosis.
        - Every 2 years in compensated cirrhosis
        - Annually in decompensated cirrhosis
    - Capsule endoscopy, a new modality for variceal screening, may be appealing as a less invasive alternative. However, its efficacy is not yet fully established. Nevertheless, capsule endoscopy remains a reasonable choice when endoscopy is high-risk.[1]
- Variceal size, classified as small, medium, or large, along with the stage of liver cirrhosis guide the recommendations for prophylaxis (see Figure 2-4).
    - Patients with medium and large varices are managed in the same way because most studies of prophylaxis grouped these classes together.
- Nonselective β-blockers have been shown to lower the risk of variceal bleeding.
    - Nonselective β-blockers act through $\beta_1$- and $\beta_2$-adrenoceptors to reduce portal blood flow.
        - $\beta_1$-adrenoceptor blockade decreases cardiac output.
        - $\beta_2$-adrenoceptor blockade causes splanchnic vasoconstriction.
        - Selective β-blockers, which only act on $\beta_1$-adrenoceptor, are much less effective.
    - β-blockers should be adjusted to the maximum tolerated dose or to maintain a resting heart rate of approximately 55 to 65 bpm.

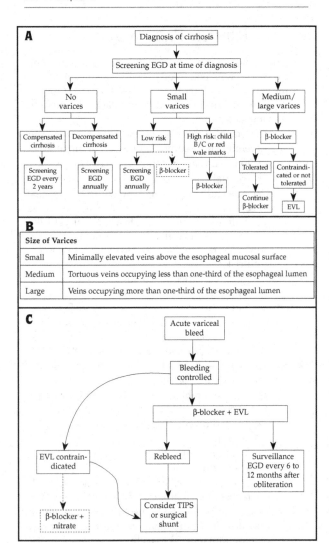

**Figure 2-4.** (A) Primary prophylaxis of variceal bleed. (B) Description of variceal size. (C) Secondary prophylaxis of variceal bleed.

- o In patients with no evidence of varices, a large randomized controlled trial showed that there was no protective effect in patients given nonselective β-blockers in the prevention of variceal development.[2]
- o When small varices are found, nonselective β-blockers may be used for the prevention of first variceal hemorrhage in patients who have an increased risk of hemorrhage as supported by the presence of Child-Pugh class B/C disease or visualized red wale marks.[3]
  - ▪ The evidence for efficacy of prophylaxis for low-risk patients with small varices is mixed.
- o In patients with medium/large varices that have not bled, β-blocker is the preferred method of treatment for the prevention of first variceal hemorrhage.
  - ▪ Among patients with medium or large varices, β-blockers reduced the rate of bleeding by more than half.[3]
- o In patients with small varices who receive β-blockers, endoscopic screening is no longer necessary.
- Prevention of variceal bleed may also be achieved by obliteration of varices with EVL.
  - o If β-blockers are contraindicated or not tolerated due to side effects, obliteration of varices using EVL can be considered.
  - o Obliteration of varices is accomplished by repeating EVL every 2 to 4 weeks. After obliteration, endoscopic surveillance is scheduled in 1 to 3 months and every 6 to 12 months thereafter.
  - o EVL may be used as primary prophylaxis of variceal bleeding, but the current data do not clearly favor endoscopic therapy over pharmacologic therapy.

- Nitrates, sclerotherapy, TIPS, and surgical shunt have no role in primary prophylaxis.

*Our patient has fully recovered after EVL, and currently has shown no evidence of bleeding in the ensuing days in the hospital. She remained on octreotide for 4 days, and an endoscopy is scheduled on the seventh hospital day prior to discharge. What should be done now to avoid a recurrent bleed?*

## SECONDARY PROPHYLAXIS

- Patients who survive an episode of acute variceal hemorrhage have a very high risk of recurrence and death and therefore should have a management plan in place before being discharged from the hospital (see Figure 2-4C).
  - Remember, the risk of recurrence is about 60% in untreated patients within 1 to 2 years of the index hemorrhage.
- The optimal treatment for preventing recurrent variceal hemorrhage is a combination of nonselective β-blocker and EVL.
  - As in primary prophylaxis, the β-blocker should be titrated to the maximal tolerated dose.
  - Adding a nitrate to the β-blocker regimen may improve efficacy of prophylaxis. This option is particularly appealing when an acute bleed has occurred in a patient who was already receiving β-blockers for primary prophylaxis and endoscopy is difficult or contraindicated. However, this combination is often poorly tolerated and rarely used.
  - In patients who have contraindication to or are unable to tolerate β-blockers due to side effects, EVL alone is performed.
    - Obliteration regimen is done as described in the above section for primary prophylaxis.

- In patients who have a recurrence of variceal hemorrhage despite combined treatment with pharmacologic and endoscopic therapy, TIPS should be considered to allow for decompression of the portal system.
- Liver transplantation provides the only definitive treatment for rebleeding because it addresses the underlying pathophysiology. Patients who are transplant candidates should be referred to a transplant center for evaluation.

*Thus far, we have focused our attention on esophageal varices, yet portal hypertension leads to pathologies at other sites, such as gastric varices, portal hypertensive gastropathy (PHG), and ectopic varices. How do we manage bleeding from these?*

# GASTRIC VARICES

- Gastric varices occur in approximately one-fifth of cirrhotic patients and account for less than 10% of cases of acute variceal bleeding.[12]
  - The lower rate of bleeding of gastric varices is explained by the following:
    - They are perfused by the short and posterior gastric veins, which have lower luminal pressure.
    - They are often decompressed by spontaneous gastrorenal shunts.
- Gastric varices are classified into 4 different categories on the basis of location, as described in Figure 2-5B.
  - GOV are simply an extension of the esophageal varices into the stomach. They are further divided into 2 groups: GOV1 and GOV2. GOV1 comprises varices that extend below the GE junction along the lesser curvature of the stomach. GOV2 describes varices that extend toward the fundus.

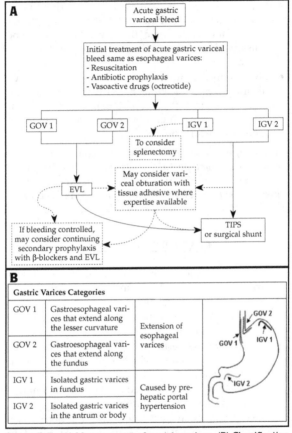

**Figure 2-5.** (A) Management of gastric varices. (B) Classification of gastric varices.

- Isolated gastric varices (IGV) are often a consequence of prehepatic portal hypertension. IGV are also divided into 2 groups: IGV1 and IGV2. IGV1 are located in the fundus, and IGV2 reside in the antrum, corpus, and around the pylorus.

- o It is important to note that IGV in the fundus (IGV1) are caused by splenic vein occlusion, in which case splenectomy may be curative.
- Due to the lower frequency of bleeding, therapy of gastric varices is not as well studied. Figure 2-5A outlines the current treatment strategies for gastric varices based on category.
- Though not established, pharmacological therapy for acute gastric variceal bleed and prophylaxis is the same as for esophageal varices.[12]
- Endoscopic treatment options for gastric varices are limited.
  - o EVL does not work well for gastric varices.
  - o Where technical expertise is available, endoscopic obliteration of gastric varices with tissue adhesives such as N-butyl-cyanoacrylate (not available for use in the United States) or 2-octyl cyanoacrylate may be attempted.
- TIPS is the therapy of choice.

# PORTAL HYPERTENSIVE GASTROPATHY

- Portal hypertension can lead to capillary dilatation of the gastric mucosa and hyperemic mucosal changes referred to as PHG.
  - o Mild PHG is characterized by a mosaic appearance of erythematous mucosa demarcated by a fine white reticular pattern.
  - o Severe PHG appears as small, red, round, and raised lesions termed *cherry red spots*.
- Approximately one-third of cirrhotic patients have PHG, and the incidence is approximately 12% per year.[8]
- PHG presents more often as a slow chronic bleed leading to iron deficiency anemia rather than an overt GI bleed.

      ○ Acute bleeding is less severe when compared to variceal bleed.
- β-blockers are also used to prevent bleeding in PHG.
  - ○ Iron supplementation is often sufficient to counteract the degree of anemia.
- TIPS may be used to manage an acute or recurrent severe bleed from PHG that is refractory to iron supplementation and β-blockers.

## ECTOPIC VARICES

TIPS can also be implemented to treat rectal and duodenal varices, although a detailed discussion of the management of these varices is beyond the scope of this chapter.

---

### Key Points
- Variceal bleeding is a devastating and potentially fatal complication of cirrhosis.
- Accurate diagnosis and timely intervention are essential for the effective treatment of variceal bleeding, which underscores the need for a high index of suspicion for patients presenting with UGIB.
- The prevalence of varices increases with the severity of cirrhosis as defined by the Child-Pugh classification, and varices develop in cirrhotic patients at a rate of 8% per year. Varices bleed at a rate of 5% to 15% per year.
- Goals of therapy include the following: volume resuscitation, control bleeding, prevent early rebleeding, and prevent complications associated with bleeding.

(continued)

## Key Points (continued)

- Resuscitative measures include hemodynamic stabilization, airway protection, coagulopathy correction, and ICU transfer.
- Antibiotic prophylaxis is of paramount importance. Antibiotics should be given to all cirrhotic patients with a UGIB, regardless of the cause of bleeding or presence of ascites.
- Control of bleeding involves a combination of pharmacologic and endoscopic therapies.
- When bleeding is refractory to pharmacologic and endoscopic therapies, TIPS and balloon tamponade can be considered as last resort interventions. Before recommending TIPS, it is important to consider the contraindications and asses the expected overall outcome. Balloon tamponade is used rarely and only as a transient bridging therapy when further definitive treatment is anticipated.
- Preventative measures should be taken as early as possible in cirrhotic patients to minimize the risk of a variceal bleeding event. The current standard of care uses careful dosing with β-blockers and periodic EGD.
- Finally, for patients who survive a variceal bleed, it is critical to have a management plan in place before discharge from the hospital, which also uses β-blockers and surveillance EGD/EVL.
- As the consulting gastroenterologist, the primary team will always look to us to accurately diagnose and manage tenuous patients during such catastrophic events. Our knowledge and understanding of pharmacologic and endoscopic therapies are therefore indispensable in giving our patients the best chance possible to survive while minimizing their risk of long-term morbidity and mortality.

# REFERENCES

1. Garcia-Tsao G, Bosch J. Management of varices and variceal hemorrhage in cirrhosis. *N Engl J Med.* 2010;362(9):823-832.

2. Groszmann RJ, Garcia-Tsao G, Bosch J, et al. Betablockers to prevent gastroesophageal varices in patients with cirrhosis. *N Engl J Med.* 2005;353(21):2254-2261.

3. Garcia-Tsao G, Sanyal AJ, Grace ND, Carey W, Practice Guidelines Committee of the American Association for the Study of Liver Diseases, Practice Parameters Committee of the American College of Gastroenterology. Prevention and management of gastroesophageal varices and variceal hemorrhage in cirrhosis. *Hepatology.* 2007;46(3):922-938.

4. Bosch J, Thabut D, Albillos A, et al. Recombinant factor VIIa for variceal bleeding in patients with advanced cirrhosis: a randomized, controlled trial. *Hepatology.* 2008;47(5):1604-1614.

5. Corley DA, Cello JP, Adkisson W, Ko WF, Kerlikowske K. Octreotide for acute esophageal variceal bleeding: a meta-analysis. *Gastroenterology.* 2001;120(4):946-954.

6. Escorsell A, Bandi JC, Andreu V, et al. Desensitization to the effects of intravenous octreotide in cirrhotic patients with portal hypertension. *Gastroenterology.* 2001;120(1):161-169.

7. Bañares R, Albillos A, Rincón D, et al. Endoscopic treatment versus endoscopic plus pharmacologic treatment for acute variceal bleeding: a meta-analysis. *Hepatology.* 2002;35(3):609-615.

8. Bosch J, D'Amico G, Garcia-Paga JC. Portal hypertension and nonsurgical management. In: Schiff ER, Sorrell MF, Maddrey WC, eds. *Diseases of the liver.* 10th ed. Philadelphia, PA: Lippincott Williams & Wilkins; 2007:419.

9. Bendtsen F, Krag A, Møller S. Treatment of acute variceal bleeding. *Dig Liver Dis.* 2008;40(5):328-336.

10. García-Pagán JC, Caca K, Bureau C, et al. Early use of TIPS in patients with cirrhosis and variceal bleeding. *N Engl J Med.* 2010;362(25):2370-2379.

11. Herrera JL. Minnesota tube placement. Practice Guideline Highlights in Gastroenterology. University of South Alabama Gastroenterology Continuing Education Site. http://usagiedu.com/minn.pdf. Accessed September 15, 2010.

12. Ryan BM, Stockbrugger RW, Ryan JM. A pathophysiologic, gastroenterologic, and radiologic approach to the management of gastric varices. *Gastroenterology.* 2004;126(4):1175-1189.

# 3

# Acute Lower Gastrointestinal Bleeding

*Hillary Tompkins, MD*
*Audrey H. Calderwood, MD*

You receive the following call from the emergency department (ED):

*We would like your advice regarding a 66-year-old man who had 2 painless bowel movements with bright red blood 4 hours ago at home and one just now while in the ED. He has had no previous episodes of bleeding. He states that he "feels okay," just a little "tired." He is still having "maroon stool with copious bright red blood and some clots." His pulse is 115 and blood pressure (BP) is 100/70. He is alert and oriented but appears very pale, and his abdomen is benign.*

Lower gastrointestinal bleeding (LGIB) is defined as bleeding beyond the ligament of Treitz and has an annual hospitalization rate of approximately 21 cases per 100,000 adults in the United States. LGIB accounts for 20% of all cases of acute GI bleeding.[1] The incidence of LGIB increases with age with a usual age range of 63 to

Lowe RC, Farraye FA.
*GI Emergencies: A Quick Reference Guide* (pp 47-60).
© 2012 Taylor & Francis Group

77 years. While it can be daunting to be faced with a de-compensating patient with active LGIB, it is reassuring to know that 75% of all LGIB stops spontaneously. The main goals in the management of LGIB are to resuscitate, diagnose the cause of the bleeding, obtain hemostasis, and prevent recurrent bleeding.

## INITIAL RESPONSE TO THE CALL

Regardless of the underlying etiology of the bleeding, there are several general recommendations you can give the primary team to help with the initial resuscitation of the patient:

- Establish large-bore intravenous (IV) access (defined as 2 peripheral IVs ≥16 gauge each).
- Resuscitation with IV fluids (normal saline [NS] or lactated ringers) and transfusion of packed red blood cells (pRBCs) as needed, taking into consideration the patient's age, comorbidities, and rate of bleeding.
- Correction of any coagulopathy.
- Strongly consider medical intensive care unit (MICU) admission if there is persistent instability in vital signs, massive or ongoing hematochezia, transfusion requirement of greater than 2 units of pRBCs, or the presence of comorbid illnesses (renal, hepatic, pulmonary, hematologic, cardiac) that put the patient at risk for complications from the LGIB or potential interventions (Table 3-1).
- If massive, ongoing bleeding associated with he-modynamic instability, consider the possibility of a brisk upper gastrointestinal bleed (UGIB).
  - o Up to 11% of patients with hematochezia have massive UGIB.[2]
  - o Perform a nasogastric (NG) tube lavage. The presence of blood in the NG tube aspirate is highly predictive of a source proximal to the ligament of Treitz[1]; however, absence of blood or bilious material in the aspirate does not exclude a possible upper source.

**Table 3-1.**

## RISK FACTORS FOR POOR OUTCOME
## IN LOWER GASTROINTESTINAL BLEEDING

- Hemodynamic instability
- Ongoing hematochezia
- Intestinal ischemia
- Comorbid illness
- Advanced age
- Bleeding while hospitalized for another process
- Use of anticoagulation or antiplatelet medications

- If the patient's abdominal exam is concerning or shows peritoneal signs, obtain a surgical consult.

## WHAT YOU NEED TO FIND OUT

While the primary team is performing its initial resuscitation, you now have the opportunity to interview and examine the patient in order to obtain the key pieces of information that will help guide your assessment of the severity of the bleeding, differential diagnosis, and initial approach to the workup. There is no substitute for evaluating the patient and assessing the primary data yourself.

Focused additional history:
- Associated symptoms: Abdominal pain, fever, weight loss, recent change in bowel habits.
- Pertinent review of systems (helps determine degree of blood loss and any sequelae): Dizziness, fatigue, chest pain, dyspnea, palpitations, etc.
- Relevant past medical history: GI, liver, cardiovascular, or renal disease; history of abdominal aortic aneurysm repair; previous GI bleeding; or endoscopic evaluations.

   o Note: There is an increased risk of complications
     and poorer outcome from LGIB with increasing
     number of medical comorbidities.
- Anticoagulation status.
- Use of nonsteroidal anti-inflammatory drugs
  (NSAIDs), aspirin, clopidogrel, and warfarin
  (Coumadin).

## PHYSICAL EXAM

- Complete set of vital signs including orthostatics to
  evaluate severity of hemodynamic compromise.
- Thorough exam with particular attention to cardiopulmonary, abdominal, and rectal exams and mental
  status.
   o Are there stigmata of chronic liver disease, such
     as spider angiomata, gynecomastia in men, or
     ascites to suggest a higher chance of a rapid
     UGIB from varices?
   o Look for anorectal pathology and gross stool
     color on rectal exam, especially if not actively
     bleeding.

## LABORATORY STUDIES

- Complete blood count (CBC), chemistries, liver
  function tests, international normalized ratio, partial
  thromboplastin time.
   o The initial CBC may not reflect the degree of
     blood loss due to hemoconcentration.
- Blood type and cross-match.

   *The patient's BP is now 110/80 with a pulse of 90
   after 1 unit of pRBCs and 1 L of NS. He continues to
   have intermittent bright red blood per rectum and is
   admitted to the MICU.*

> ## Key Points
> - Adequate IV access and aggressive resuscitation are essential in the initial management of LGIB.
> - Orthostatic vital signs can help determine degree of blood loss and effectiveness of resuscitation.
> - Initial hematocrit and hemoglobin values may not reflect the degree of blood loss, so you must reassess on an ongoing basis once resuscitation has begun.

## DIAGNOSTIC TESTS TO CONSIDER AND PERFORM

After initial resuscitation, the main goal is to diagnose the source of the bleeding (Table 3-2). The patient's age, comorbidities, and previous or recent colonoscopies or interventions will help prioritize your differential diagnosis and, thus, your workup. If a brisk UGIB is suspected, then an esophagogastroduodenoscopy (EGD) should be performed prior to colonoscopy. In addition to the 11% of patients initially suspected of having LGIB actually having an upper source, an additional 10% to 20% of patients presenting with LGIB can be found to have a small bowel source of bleeding.[2] While no large, controlled trials have demonstrated a clear advantage of a particular diagnostic strategy for presumed LGIB, the following summarizes diagnostic tests to consider in your workup.

### Colonoscopy
- The initial test of choice to evaluate for a structural cause.
- Has the advantage of being both diagnostic and potentially therapeutic.
- Diagnostic yield ranges from 75% to 100% based on clinical studies.[3]
- Optimal timing of performing colonoscopy is not well supported by evidence in the literature, but most recommend performing within 12 to 48 hours depending on severity and persistence of bleeding.

**Table 3-2.**

## SOURCES FOR LOWER GASTROINTESTINAL BLEEDING IN ORDER OF FREQUENCY

| SOURCE | FREQUENCY (%) | COMMENTS/CLINICAL PEARLS |
|---|---|---|
| Diverticular disease | 15 to 55 | Acute painless hematochezia, arterial bleeding, most resolve spontaneously but 10% to 40% will have recurrent bleeding.[4,5] Incidence increases with increasing age. Right-sided tend to bleed more than left-sided. About 20% will require intervention. |
| Angio-dysplasia | 3 to 37 | Venous bleeding, usually multiple, most do not bleed. Incidence increases with increasing age. Usually episodic bleeding that increases in setting of anticoagulation or coagulopathy and likely in patients with end-stage renal disease. If no active bleeding or signs of recent bleeding (eg, visible vessel, clot) on colonoscopy, consider alternate bleeding source. |
| Colitis: ischemic, infectious, inflammatory, radiation induced | 6 to 22 | Ischemic—acute onset of mild abdominal pain followed by hematochezia or bloody diarrhea. History and physical can often reveal cause. Is associated with an increased risk of mortality. Treat underlying cause. |

*(continued)*

**Table 3-2. (continued)**

## SOURCES FOR LOWER GASTROINTESTINAL BLEEDING IN ORDER OF FREQUENCY

| SOURCE | FREQUENCY (%) | COMMENTS/CLINICAL PEARLS |
|--------|---------------|--------------------------|
| Colitis: ischemic, infectious, inflammatory, radiation induced | 6 to 22 | Radiation telangiectasia—9 to 14 months post-radiation therapy for abdominal or pelvic cancers. Generally treated with repeated sessions with APC. |
| Colonic neoplasia | 8 to 19 | Usually on the left side or polyps >1 cm. |
| Post-polypectomy | 2 to 6[5] | Most frequent complication. Can be acute or delayed and seen at 14 days postprocedure. Review colonoscopy report (largest polyp removed most likely to bleed) and inform gastroenterologist of complication. |
| Anorectal: hemorrhoids, varices | 4 to 9 | Usually intermittent and low volume. Can be treated by ligation with bands. |
| Dieulafoy's lesion | Rare | Acute, overt, arterial bleeding from a vessel that protrudes through normal mucosa. Most case reports are of a lesion in the rectum. Best mode of treatment not established. |

*(continued)*

**Table 3-2. (continued)**

## SOURCES FOR LOWER GASTROINTESTINAL BLEEDING IN ORDER OF FREQUENCY

| SOURCE | FREQUENCY (%) | COMMENTS/ CLINICAL PEARLS |
|---|---|---|
| UGIB | 0 to 11 | Accounts for up to 11% of massive hematochezia. |
| Small bowel bleeding: neoplasia, inflammatory bowel disease, angiodysplasia, Meckel's diverticulum | 2 to 9 | May be suspected based on patient age and history. Should be considered if evaluation does not reveal another source. |

- If the patient has stopped bleeding and is hemo-dynamically stable, colonoscopy can be pursued more electively during the admission after a colonic purge. Series have shown a trend toward higher diagnostic and therapeutic yields when colonoscopy is performed earlier without a significant difference in mortality.[3]
- Terminal ileal intubation should always be attempted because this can help localize the bleeding site if no specific source is identified.
- Very safe to perform after appropriate resuscitation. Complication rate ranges from 0.2% to 2% in published case series.[3]
- For patients with severe bleeding, rapid colonic purge can be pursued, which can improve visualization and diagnostic yield.[6,7]

- o Give 4 to 6 L of a polyethylene glycol solution over 2 to 3 hours.
- o Lavage through NG tube may be necessary; however, avoid this in patients who are at a high risk of aspiration.
- o Can give metoclopramide 10 mg IV or PO (oral) at the start of the purge to promote gastric emptying and prevent nausea.
- o Ideal to perform colonoscopy as soon as possible after purge is completed.

## Angiography

- The only radiographic modality that is both diagnostic and therapeutic.
- Requires active bleeding (rate $\geq$0.5 to 1.0 mL/min) to detect extravasation.
- Most useful for massive bleeding in which hemodynamic instability precludes colonoscopy or when bleeding persists and colonoscopy is nondiagnostic.
- Diagnostic yield ranges from 25% to 78% in clinical series.[3,8]
- Can localize bleeding for surgery or provide treatment with embolization materials with success rates reported to be 70% to 90%.[1]
- Most likely to be positive with diverticular bleeding.
- Potential complications include contrast allergy, renal failure, hematomas, bleeding, embolism, vascular dissections, and bowel infarction (most common major complication).

## Radionuclide Scintigraphy/Nuclear Medicine Bleeding Scans

- Threshold for detection of bleeding is slower than for angiography (0.1 to 0.4 mL/min).
- Purely diagnostic without therapeutic capabilities.

- Most useful in localizing slow, intermittent bleeding that continues after a nondiagnostic colonoscopy prior to angiography or surgery; however, sensitivity and specificity in localization of bleeding is variable in the literature. Often only localizes bleeding to a general area of the GI tract.
- Review of studies since 1998 revealed a 66% accuracy of a positive test.[3]
- Often used as a screening test prior to angiography because a positive scan increases the success of a mesenteric angiogram.
- Need to facilitate urgent angiography in anticipation of a positive scan.

*Computed Tomography Scan*

- Along with abdominal plain film, initial test of choice if you suspect perforation or obstruction.
- Multidetector row computed tomography (CT) allows arterial images that can show contrast extravasation in the setting of slow bleeding rates and thus assist with localization with a yield ranging from 25% to 95% in the literature.[3]
- May show colonic thickening and stranding that support a diagnosis of colitis, whether ischemic, infectious, or inflammatory. While CT is not reliable in differentiating among the possible causes of colitis, the distribution of colonic changes may alter the likelihood of certain diseases.

If bleeding persists and an evaluation of the upper GI tract and colon has not revealed a source, evaluation of the small bowel for a bleeding source should be considered. Evaluation can be done with enteroscopy, capsule endoscopy, CT, or magnetic resonance enterography depending on the availability and expertise of your facility.

---

### *Key Points*

- If brisk persistent hematochezia with hemodynamic instability, consider the possibility that this is a UGIB, and perform urgent EGD.
- Always consent for an upper endoscopy at time of consent for colonoscopy to allow you the option to complete evaluation for upper GI source if colonoscopy is unrevealing.
- The primary roles of colonoscopy are to diagnose the source of bleeding and provide hemostasis where possible, but it can also be very helpful in excluding causes and localizing the site of bleeding even if a specific etiology is not found.
- Rapid colonic purge includes 3 to 6 L of a polyethylene glycol solution given over 2 hours until the patient is clear from below. Remember the risk of aspiration in those with poor mental status if given via NG tube.

---

*After colonic purge with 4 L of polyethylene glycol solution, an urgent colonoscopy is performed at the bedside in the MICU. Fresh blood is seen in the left colon, and multiple diverticula are noted throughout the descending and sigmoid colon without a culprit bleeding site. There is no blood seen in the terminal ileum.*

## THERAPEUTIC OPTIONS IN ACUTE LOWER GASTROINTESTINAL BLEEDING

The main goal of therapy is to obtain hemostasis and prevent recurrent bleeding. During colonoscopy, several endoscopic techniques are available to provide hemostasis. In cases of LGIB, endoscopic therapy is applied in 10% to 40%, and hemostasis is achieved in 50% to 100% of the cases.[3]

## Colonoscopy

- Thermal coagulation with bipolar or monopolar electrocoagulation, heater probe, or argon plasma coagulation (APC) can be used.
- The risk of perforation is higher in the right colon compared to the left and lowest with use of APC.
- Injection of vasoconstrictors such as epinephrine at 1:10,000 dilution can also be used in 1- to 2-mL aliquots in 4 quadrants around the source of bleeding to obtain temporary hemostasis and improve visibility.
- Hemostasis using metallic clips and band ligation can also be performed.
- There are variable data on the immediate and long-term control of diverticular bleeding with colonoscopic techniques. Use of epinephrine injection and electrocoagulation in 3 case series provided immediate control of the hemorrhage in 25% to 86% but was associated with early re-bleeding rates of 25% to 38%. Use of hemoclips controlled 100% of diverticular bleeding in a single series.[5]
- Angiodysplasias: Best treated with APC or other form of electrocautery. Use of clips has only been described in case reports.

## Angiography With Transcatheter Embolization

- Offers success in 70% to 90% of cases.[1]
- Most useful in diverticular bleeds.
- Fifteen percent failure rate to control diverticular bleeding based on one meta-analysis.[8]
- Useful for persistent hematochezia from diverticular bleed when colonoscopy can not localize the source.
- Ischemia has become a rare complication with development of new microcatheters and embolization techniques but still remains the most common major complication.

# SURGERY

- Consider if persistent and life-threatening bleeding or recurrent bleeding despite endoscopic and radiographic therapies.
- Treatment of choice for bleeding from neoplasia.
- Amount of blood needed for initial resuscitation in first 24 hours corresponds with likelihood of requiring surgery. In one single-center review of diverticular bleeding, the receipt of more than 4 units pRBCs was associated with a 60% likelihood of going to surgery.[9]
- Directed segmental resection is the treatment of choice when surgery is necessary.
- Multiple clinical series have shown a decreased morbidity and mortality if the site of bleeding is localized prior to surgical intervention.

---

### Key Points

- There are multiple options for endoscopic hemostasis: thermal coagulation, injection of vasoconstrictors, and metallic clips. No studies have shown superiority of one over the other.
- Perforation risk is highest in the right colon and cecum.
- Surgery is considered only if all other diagnostic and therapeutic options are unsuccessful.

---

*The patient has more hematochezia, and his heart rate increases. He is sent for an urgent tagged nuclear medicine bleeding scan with angiography back-up as needed. The bleeding scan is positive in the left upper quadrant, and the patient proceeds to angiography. Active extravasation is seen, and embolization is successful at stopping the bleeding.*

# REFERENCES

1. Barnet J, Messmann H. Diagnosis and management of lower gastrointestinal bleeding. *Nat Rev Gastroenterol Hepatol.* 2009;6:637-646.

2. Jensen DM, Machicado GA. Diagnosis and treatment of severe hematochezia. The role of urgent colonoscopy after purge. *Gastroenterology.* 1988;95:1569-1574.

3. Strate LL, Naumann CR. The role of colonoscopy and radiological procedures in the management of acute lower intestinal bleeding. *Clin Gastroenterol Hepatol.* 2010;8:333-343.

4. Adams JB, Margolin DA. Management of diverticular hemorrhage. *Clin Colon Rectal Surg.* 2009;22:181-185.

5. Davila RE, Rajan E, Adler DG, et al. ASGE guideline: the role of endoscopy in the patient with lower-GI bleeding. *Gastrointest Endosc.* 2005;62:656-660.

6. Elta GH. Urgent colonoscopy for acute lower-GI bleeding. *Gastrointest Endosc.* 2004;59:402-408.

7. Longstreth GF. Epidemiology and outcome of patients hospitalized with acute lower gastrointestinal hemorrhage: a population-based study. *Am J Gastroenterol.* 1997;92:419-424.

8. Zuccaro G. Management of the adult patient with acute lower gastrointestinal bleeding. *Am J Gastroenterol.* 1998;93(8):1202-1208.

9. McGuire HH Jr. Bleeding colonic diverticula. A reappraisal of natural history and management. *Ann Surg.* 1994;220:653-656.

# 4

# Evaluation of Acute Abdominal Pain

*Joseph Feuerstein, MD*
*M. Michael Wolfe, MD*

You receive the following call from the emergency department (ED):

*A 23-year-old woman has been brought in by her friend, writhing in pain. She developed acute diffuse abdominal pain 1 hour earlier. Her exam is notable for fever (102°F), a heart rate of 112, and a blood pressure of 110/76. She is found curled up in the fetal position, with diffuse abdominal tenderness and guarding on physical examination. Lab tests are pending. We would like you to help us in evaluating this patient. As noted in* **Cope's Early Diagnosis of the Acute Abdomen,** *"abdominal pain is one of the most common conditions that calls for prompt diagnosis and treatment."[1]*

The most important issues to consider in a patient with severe abdominal pain are as follows:

- Is this a "surgical" abdomen?
- Is this a life-threatening condition that needs immediate nonsurgical therapy?
- Is this a less serious condition that can be evaluated in a less urgent fashion?

Lowe RC, Farraye FA.
*GI Emergencies: A Quick Reference Guide* (pp 61-72).
© 2012 Taylor & Francis Group

## WHAT IS THE INITIAL WORKUP?

- The most important aspect in determining the cause of any patient presenting with abdominal pain is a thorough history. While the differential diagnosis of abdominal pain includes numerous etiologies, a careful history can significantly reduce a long list to a few likely causes. Though we all have been taught to evaluate pain using the PQRST mnemonic (provoking or palliating factors, quality, radiation, severity, timing), a skilled clinician must recognize the importance of each of these features and know the patterns associated with common and uncommon disorders.

- Pain must be characterized as to when it started, precipitating factors, and maneuvers that alleviate the pain.

- Distinguishing acute (minutes to hours) versus chronic pain (months to years) is essential in narrowing the differential diagnosis. Cope comments, "The general rule can be laid down that majority of severe abdominal pains that ensue in patients who have been previously fairly well, and that last as long as 6 hours, are caused by conditions of surgical import."[1] Similarly, the severity of the pain must be established. A pain scale of 1 to 10 can be helpful; however, in one isolated moment, the pain may be reported as mild, but as time progresses, it may worsen or stabilize. Thus, it is important to reassess the patient frequently in order to monitor for changes in the severity or quality of pain.

- It should be noted that patients taking corticosteroids may have only mild abdominal pain despite severe disease as the inflammatory response may be suppressed by the corticosteroids. In such a patient, even mild abdominal pain should be evaluated thoroughly.

- The nature and location of the pain can further narrow the source:

- Colicky or intermittent crampy pain may suggest bowel obstruction; the pain of renal colic will also wax and wane while "biliary colic" is typically not "colicky," but more a constant unremitting pain.[2]
- Right upper quadrant pain radiating around to the scapula often indicates pancreatic or biliary disease. This pain may also be described as postprandial, reaching a crescendo over time, then subsiding after 1 to 2 hours.[2]
- In contrast, sharp epigastric pain radiating to the back makes pancreatitis or perforated peptic ulcer more likely. The pain of pancreatitis is often worse when the patient lies supine and improves with sitting forward.
- "Tearing" pain is more classically associated with a vascular event like a ruptured thoracic or abdominal aortic aneurysm, although only a minority of patients use these descriptors.
- Pain from an inflammatory process tends to be sharp and continuous, with tenderness on deep palpation over the involved organ, as in appendicitis or diverticulitis. Inflammation, however, may begin with referred pain to a different area of the abdomen that, over time, usually localizes over the area of inflammation. Cholecystitis may begin with visceral epigastric pain that shifts to the right upper quadrant when the parietal peritoneum becomes inflamed, while appendicitis may begin with visceral pain in the mid abdomen before moving to the right lower quadrant.
- Lower quadrant pain is more difficult to narrow down and can be associated with many gastrointestinal (GI) and non-GI causes. In young women especially, the differential for non-GI causes is quite broad, including salpingitis, ectopic pregnancy, ruptured ovarian cyst, etc. See Table 4-1 for a more detailed differential diagnosis of the causes of pain based on location.

**Table 4-1.**

## COMMON CAUSES OF ACUTE ABDOMINAL PAIN

| LOCATION | DIFFERENTIAL DIAGNOSIS |
|---|---|
| Right upper quadrant | Cholelithiasis, cholecystitis, cholangitis, biliary dyskinesia, liver abscess/cyst, Fitz-Hugh-Curtis syndrome, pneumonia/empyema |
| Right lower quadrant | Appendicitis, diverticulitis, inflammatory bowel disease (IBD), mesenteric adenitis, nephrolithiasis, salpingitis, pregnancy/ectopic pregnancy |
| Epigastric | Dyspepsia, gastroesophageal reflux disease (GERD), peptic ulcer disease, gastritis, pancreatitis, gastroenteritis, eosinophilic gastritis, myocardial infarction |
| Left upper quadrant | Splenic infarction, splenic abscess, pneumonia/empyema |
| Left lower quadrant | Diverticulitis, volvulus, IBD, constipation, nephrolithiasis, salpingitis, pregnancy/ectopic pregnancy |
| Diffuse | Intestinal ischemia, bowel obstruction, malabsorption, irritable bowel syndrome, peritonitis, abdominal migraines |
| Diffuse—non-GI causes | Abdominal aortic aneurysm, diabetic ketoacidosis, hypercalcemia, adrenal insufficiency, testicular torsion, pyelonephritis, ovarian cyst rupture, mittelschmerz, familial Mediterranean fever, acute porphyria, sickle cell crisis |

    ○ The pain of renal colic is severe and is usually localized to the flank and upper abdomen on the affected side. If the stone is in the lower portion of the ureter, pain may be referred to the ipsilateral testicle in men and to the labium in women.

- Precipitating factors and some associated symptoms can help delineate the etiology of the pain. Pain increasing with movement, coughing, laughing, or sneezing may be peritoneal in origin, which should warrant an urgent surgical consultation. Pain worsened by food may point toward a biliary source, although GERD and peptic ulcer symptoms may also be exacerbated by food intake. Pain associated with the midpoint of the menstrual cycle is possibly mittelschmerz, while episodic pain during menses should make endometriosis a consideration. While fevers indicate a worrisome pathology, the presence of nausea, vomiting, diarrhea, and weight loss are all important but are uncommonly helpful in locating the source of pain.

- Medications can also be the cause of the patient's acute abdominal pain, and a thorough medication history, including herbal supplements, can further narrow the differential diagnosis.

- A patient's comorbidities may help determine the diagnosis of pain. Prior surgery places a patient at increased risk for obstruction from adhesion formation. A patient with long-standing diabetes with associated complications is at risk of developing gastroparesis with episodic severe nausea and vomiting. Both Crohn's disease and ulcerative colitis usually manifest as recurrent flares characterized by abdominal pain; increased stool frequency; mucus; hematochezia; and, on occasion, fevers, chills, nausea, and vomiting.

## PHYSICAL EXAMINATION

After a thorough history, the differential diagnosis can be further narrowed by a detailed physical exam to support or refute initial diagnostic considerations.

- Inspection: Is the patient writhing in pain or relatively comfortable? Keep in mind, however, that even a comfortable-appearing patient may have peritonitis. Inspecting for downward displacement of the umbilicus beyond 1 cm from the midpoint between xiphoid and symphysis pubis (Tanyol sign) may be an indication of underlying ascites, whereas upward displacement is more consistent with pregnancy or a pelvic mass lesion. Abnormal patterns of respirations hint toward an inflammatory process. During respiration, areas of inflammation in the abdomen will remain motionless. In contrast, in pneumonia, the abdomen moves freely, while the lower chest is restricted. Also, surgical scars, if present, indicate an increased risk of adhesion-induced obstruction.
- Vital signs should be evaluated for tachycardia and especially orthostatic hypotension in any patient with blood loss, complaints of dizziness, or following a syncopal event.[3]
- Skin: Examine for stigmata of liver pathology or signs of bleeding from intraperitoneal or retroperitoneal etiologies.
  - The presence of spider angiomata on the neck or upper chest is most indicative of portal hypertension; other stigmata include palmar erythema, Dupuytren's contractures, gynecomastia, Terry's nails, and testicular atrophy.
  - Grey Turner's sign (ecchymoses of the flank) or Cullen's sign (umbilical ecchymosis) may be consistent with hemorrhagic pancreatitis; however, it has very poor specificity, occurring in ectopic pregnancy and retroperitoneal hemorrhage.
  - The abdominal venous pattern may suggest portal hypertension (severe engorgement may present with caput medusae) or inferior vena cava obstruction (linear vein engorgement along one or both flanks).

- Abdominal exam: Auscultation of the abdomen is necessary to determine the presence or lack of bowel sounds. Occasionally, high-pitched rushing bowel sounds may indicate an obstruction. Otherwise, the presence of bowel sounds usually excludes a diagnosis of intestinal obstruction. Absent bowel sounds in a patient with an acute abdomen are associated with severe peritonitis. The abdomen should also be auscultated for abdominal bruits, which would increase the likelihood of an ischemic etiology for pain. Percussion should be performed to assess for free air (resonant), distention (tympanic), ascites (shifting dullness), and peritoneal signs. In cases of peritonitis, the abdominal wall is often rigid and immobile even with respiration. Palpation should be done in all quadrants, first lightly and then more deeply. Involuntary guarding and rebound (the springing back of stretched abdominal wall musculature that, if inflamed, triggers pain, also known as Blumberg's sign) can be helpful. Note that shaking the patient gently, asking the patient to cough, or percussing the abdomen can also bring out the pain of peritonitis, obviating the need for the more painful "rebound" test.
- Both hepatomegaly and splenomegaly can be assessed with deep palpation.
- Digital rectal exam can be helpful in eliciting pain from lower abdominal organs (retrocecal appendix) and in revealing melena or hematochezia.
- Different maneuvers can also be performed to further narrow the differential.
  - Carnett's sign: Ask the patient while lying down to lift his or her head off the bed while tucking chin to chest, thereby creating voluntary guarding by contracting the abdominal musculature. If there is unchanged or worsening pain on palpation (ie, a positive sign), it indicates a musculoskeletal etiology, such as rectus sheath

hemorrhage. If there is no pain or the pain is decreased in intensity, a visceral cause is more likely.[4] Also, if the pain can be elicited by palpation in a small localized area (ie, with one finger), the likelihood of abdominal wall pain is increased.

o Murphy's sign: Palpate beneath the ribs in the right upper quadrant and have the patient take a deep breath. If the patient does not complete the inspiration due to pain, this is a positive sign, indicating inflammation in the right upper quadrant, most often associated with cholecystitis.[2]

o Rovsing's sign: Palpate in the left iliac fossa; if this triggers referred pain in the right iliac fossa, it is a positive test and should make the examiner concerned about appendicitis. The better test for appendicitis though is palpation at McBurney's point—pain on palpation 1.5 to 2 inches from the anterior spinous process of the ileum in a straight line down to the umbilicus.

o Obturator test: With the patient supine, flex the thigh and rotate inward. If this is positive only on the right, it may indicate appendicitis. Overall though, the test is useful in evaluating for inflammatory processes in the lower abdomen.

o Psoas sign: If there is inflammation around the iliopsoas muscle, then the thigh is usually found flexed as the position of comfort. If inflammation is milder, having the patient lay on the opposite side of the presumed inflamed focus and extending the thigh on the affected side fully will elicit either referred pain or pain from direct inflammation of the muscle.

o Shifting dullness can be used to assess for ascites. Note that flank dullness alone is not sufficient. There must be a shift to confirm the presence of intra-abdominal fluid. A fluid wave is also helpful, although it is positive only when a large amount of fluid is present.[4]

# LABORATORY TESTING

Laboratory testing should be limited to support or refute the leading differential diagnosis that was formed from the history and physical. A scattershot approach without an underlying hypothesis can lead to diagnostic error as abnormal values can be followed even when they are inconsistent with the clinical picture.

- A complete blood count (CBC) with differential should be checked on any patient in whom an infectious etiology or hemorrhage is suspected. Additionally, the differential on the CBC may be the only clue to diseases such as eosinophilic esophagitis, eosinophilic gastroenteritis, and nematode infestation. In cases of GI bleeding, the hematocrit may take up to 48 hours to fully equilibrate. It is still useful to check, but the magnitude of blood loss must be evaluated clinically as well. The platelet count is useful because a low platelet count may indicate underlying portal HTN from liver disease, while an elevated count is seen in inflammatory states and with iron deficiency anemia.

- Electrolytes and blood urea nitrogen/creatinine can be helpful in cases of diarrhea and complications of diseases, such as the hepatorenal syndrome.

- Aminotransferases, alkaline phosphatase, bilirubin, and markers of liver synthetic function (international normalized ratio, albumin) should be ordered in patients with presumed liver pathology.

- Amylase and lipase should be checked together for pancreatitis as elevations in both of these tests are more sensitive and specific for pancreatitis than either test alone.

- Serum lactate can be helpful in cases of acute ischemia, especially when a metabolic acidosis is present; however, chronic mesenteric ischemia may not have an elevated blood lactate, and therefore this test cannot exclude such a diagnosis.

# IMAGING

Imaging serves as a key diagnostic modality in evaluating acute abdominal pain because laboratory tests are rarely diagnostic of abdominal pathology.

- A plain abdominal x-ray (kidneys, ureters, and bladder [KUB]) still has utility in a computed tomography (CT)-centric world, as it can be rapidly performed and uses little radiation. However, its utility should not be overstated. In a study of more than 1000 KUB exams in a Canadian ED, the study was diagnostic in 80 cases, with bowel obstruction, perforation (free air), and renal stones being the major diagnostic categories observed. Thus, if obstruction or perforation is suspected, an abdominal film may be of value (because noncontrast CT has replaced other modalities for the diagnosis of renal stones).[5]

- CT scan with oral and intravenous contrast is most useful in the patient presenting with diffuse abdominal pain. Abdominal KUB is of little utility when a CT scan is readily available. A CT has a sensitivity of 89% and a specificity of 77% for serious conditions in patients presenting with acute abdominal pain.[6]

- Ultrasound should be used if a hepatobiliary source is suspected because it has a sensitivity of 94% and specificity of 78% for acute cholecystitis.[7] A meta-analysis evaluating the utility of either clinical findings or laboratory testing to rule out acute cholecystitis found that neither alone or combined had strong enough likelihood ratios to rule in or rule out acute cholecystitis without ultrasound imaging.[2]

- The sensitivity of ultrasound in the evaluation of acute abdominal pain for an urgent diagnosis was 70%.[8]

- One study looking at patients presenting with acute abdominal pain using a strategy of ultrasonography first followed by CT resulted in a combined sensitivity of 94% for establishing a diagnosis.[8]

- Emergent surgery/exploratory laparotomy should be considered for any patient with physical exam findings concerning for peritonitis.

## Key Points:

- Common radiation patterns of pain should be recognized and taught to trainees:
  - pancreatic pain → mid-back
  - biliary pain → right scapula
  - renal stones in the distal ureter → ipsilateral testis or labium
  - peptic ulcer → left or right lower quadrant (not truly radiation, but due to leakage of inflammatory fluid down the paracolic gutters)
- Carnett's sign (worsening of pain with tensing of the abdominal muscles) may be useful in indicating a musculoskeletal cause for abdominal pain
- The pain of peritonitis can be elicited with "rebound testing," but pain with percussion, with cough, or with gentle shaking of the patient can also reveal peritonitis with less patient discomfort. Remember that a patient who is "writhing" in pain typically does not have peritonitis—such patients typically lie still and resist movement.
- The term *colic* refers to a waxing and waning pain, such as that seen with bowel obstruction. Biliary colic is a misnomer, as this pain is typically constant after building to a plateau, then resolving after 1 to 3 hours.
- Corticosteroid use can decrease the intensity of abdominal pain, so abdominal pain in these patients must be investigated thoroughly.
- Imaging should be targeted to the most likely cause of pain. Abdominal plain films can reveal perforation, bowel, obstruction, and occasionally renal stones; ultrasound reveals hepatobiliary or renal pathology; and CT is best for visualizing solid organ disease, bowel inflammation, and intra-abdominal fluid collections/abscesses.

# REFERENCES

1. Silen W. *Cope's Early Diagnosis of the Acute Abdomen*. 20th ed. New York, NY: Oxford University Press; 2000.
2. Trowbridge RL, Rutkowski NK, Shojania KG. Does this patient have acute cholecystitis? *JAMA*. 2003;289:80-86.
3. McGee S, Abernethy WB 3rd, Simel DL. The rational clinical examination. Is this patient hypovolemic? *JAMA*. 1999;281:1022-1029.
4. Orient J. *Sapira's Art & Science of Bedside Diagnosis*. 3rd ed. Philadelphia, PA: Lippincott Williams & Wilkins; 2005:443-464.
5. Eisenberg RL, Heineken P, Hedgcock MW, Federle M, Goldberg HI. Evaluation of plain abdominal radiographs in the diagnosis of acute abdominal pain. *Ann Surg*. 1983;197(4):464-469.
6. Rosen MP, Sands DZ, Longmaid HE 3rd, Reynolds KF, Wagner M, Raptopoulos V. Impact of abdominal CT on the management of patients presenting to the emergency department with acute abdominal pain. *AJR Am J Roentgenol*. 2000;174:1391-1396.
7. Shea JA, Berlin JA, Escarce JJ, et al. Revised estimates of diagnostic test sensitivity and specificity in suspected biliary tract disease. *Arch Intern Med*. 1994;154:2573-2581.
8. Laméris W, van Randen A, van Es HW, et al. Imaging strategies for detection of urgent conditions in patients with acute abdominal pain: diagnostic accuracy study. *BMJ*. 2009;338:b2431.

# 5

# Bowel Obstruction and Pseudo-Obstruction

*Joann Kwah, MD*
*Wanda P. Blanton, MD*

You receive the following call from the emergency department (ED):

*A patient was brought in from his nursing home with a past medical history significant for advanced Parkinson's disease. He is sent here because the staff noted worsening abdominal distension and altered mental status. They also noted that the patient has not had a bowel movement in 5 days. Enemas and oral laxatives were given over the past few days, but the patient still did not have a bowel movement. An abdominal x-ray shows massive colonic distension with a classic inverted U-shaped appearance suspicious for volvulus.*

## COLONIC VOLVULUS

- Volvulus occurs when the large bowel twists on its own mesenteric axis, causing partial or complete obstruction and congestion of the blood supply that can progress to infarction or gangrene.[1] Clinical

Lowe RC, Farraye FA.
*GI Emergencies: A Quick Reference Guide* (pp 73-90).
© 2012 Taylor & Francis Group

presentation can be acute or subacute, with the most common symptom and sign being abdominal distension.

- Volvulus accounts for less than 5% of cases of large bowel obstruction. Endoscopic decompression is usually attempted for sigmoid volvulus in the absence of peritoneal signs or perforation.[1]
- Most common populations at risk for volvulus are elderly patients, patients from chronic care facilities, and patients with severe neurological disease or psychiatric illness.[2]
- Special populations: Sigmoid volvulus is the most common cause of intestinal obstruction in pregnancy, accounting for nearly 45% of all intestinal obstructions in this group of women.
- Less common populations at risk: Patients with Hirschsprung's or Chagas disease are also at higher risk for colonic volvulus.

## WHAT ARE YOUR NEXT STEPS?

- This condition requires urgent attention because the bowel is at high risk for infarction and perforation if not treated promptly.
- Determine, from talking to the ED physician, whether there is evidence of ischemic complications, such as peritoneal signs or free air on the abdominal x-ray. Regardless of the signs and symptoms, patients with a clinical suspicion of volvulus should be evaluated by the surgical consult team.
- As you are on your way to the hospital, your initial thought process should include the following:
  - If this is a volvulus, in what part of the colon is it located?
    - A sigmoid volvulus is more amenable to endoscopic decompression compared to a volvulus in the cecum or transverse colon, which is usually managed surgically.

- Although endoscopic decompression has been described for cecal volvulus and transverse colon volvulus, the success rate is much lower.
  - If this is not a volvulus, what else could be causing the obstruction?
    - Mechanical obstruction is less common in the large bowel than the small bowel, with approximately 10% to 15% of bowel obstruction cases involving the colon. Common causes of colonic obstruction include the following:
      - Colon cancer
      - Diverticular disease with stricture
      - Fecal impaction
      - Anastomotic stricture
- Once you are evaluating the patient:
  - Additional relevant history: Any previous history of volvulus that was managed nonoperatively? Patients with a prior history of volvulus who did not have definitive surgical treatment are at high risk for recurrence. Other pertinent history includes chronic constipation, previous abdominal surgeries, or pelvic tumors, which are risk factors for volvulus.
  - Physical exam
    - Abdominal exam will reveal a markedly distended abdomen in more than 50% of patients.
    - Ensure that surgery has been called to evaluate the patient.
    - Although not sensitive or specific for colonic ischemia, additional pertinent exam findings would include the following:
      - Vital signs demonstrating tachycardia or hypotension.
      - Rectal exam with bloody stool may suggest ischemic compromise to the colon.

- o Laboratory studies
  - ▪ Complete blood count (CBC), chemistries, and lactic acid can be helpful, as leukocytosis and a metabolic acidosis may be present.
- o Imaging
  - ▪ Abdominal x-rays are diagnostic in 60% to 75% of cases. Clinical pearl: Review the films with the radiologist. You can often get a better sense of how certain he or she is of the diagnosis and whether additional imaging would be helpful.
  - ▪ Appearance of a sigmoid volvulus on abdominal x-ray:
    - □ Inverted U-shaped appearance of the distended sigmoid colon that has formed a closed loop obstruction (Figure 5-1). Note the loss of haustra.
    - □ Radiologists may also refer to this radiologic finding as a "coffee-bean sign."
    - □ Lack of stool and air in the rectal vault implies an obstruction versus an ileus.
- o If imaging does not confirm a volvulus, consider the following additional imaging modalities:
  - ▪ Whirl sign on abdominal computed tomography (CT) represents the twisting of engorged vessels and mesentery radiating from the axis of bowel rotation (Figure 5-2).
  - ▪ Although water-soluble contrast enemas have been used to diagnose a colonic volvulus, we favor CT because it can reveal other potential etiologies for abdominal pain and is less invasive.

## MANAGEMENT RECOMMENDATIONS

- Medical management should include the following:
  - o NPO (nothing by mouth), volume resuscitation, and correction of metabolic derangements.

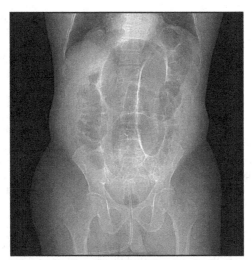

**Figure 5-1.** Sigmoid volvulus. (Reprinted with permission of Avneesh Gupta, MD.)

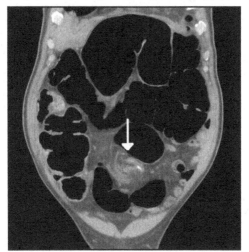

**Figure 5-2.** Whirl sign on CT (white arrow). (Reprinted with permission of Avneesh Gupta, MD.)

Consider nasogastric (NG) tube for proximal gut decompression if patient has upper gastrointestinal (GI) symptoms, such as nausea or vomiting.

o Consider intravenous (IV) broad-spectrum antibiotics to cover anaerobic and aerobic bacteria if there are signs of colonic ischemia.

o Review of medications to avoid any agents that may decrease GI motility including opiates, calcium-channel blockers, and anticholinergics.

- Sigmoid volvulus: In the absence of peritoneal signs, endoscopic decompression should be attempted urgently as it has a success rate as high as 80%.[3]

  o Minimize air insufflation with advancement of the endoscope.

  o As you approach the volvulus, you will see twisted colonic mucosa. Assess mucosa for signs of ischemia and whether it is safe to proceed with advancement of the endoscope.

  o If there are no signs of perforation or ischemia, gently advance the endoscope through the twisted segment. Then, suction fluid and air contents as the endoscope is withdrawn.

  o If ischemic mucosa is visualized on endoscopy, decompression should be abandoned and surgical resection should be performed.

  o Once decompression has been achieved, a rectal tube can be placed proximal to the point of the decompressed volvulus for 24 to 72 hours.

  o A follow-up abdominal x-ray to check for, or rule-out, free air is performed following the endoscopic procedure.

- Surgeons should be involved early on (ie, before endoscopy is performed) because these patients may need urgent surgical intervention if the sigmoid volvulus cannot be decompressed endoscopically or if there is evidence of colonic ischemia.

  o In general, endoscopic decompression is considered a temporizing measure until definitive surgical treatment (cecopexy or bowel resection) to avoid recurrence of the volvulus, which can be as high as 50% after decompression.[1]

o Colonic volvulus in the cecum or transverse colon is usually managed surgically. The success rate of endoscopic decompression is much less.

---

### Key Points to Sigmoid Volvulus

- This is a medical emergency and should be evaluated and treated as soon as possible to avoid complications of colonic ischemia. If you are called to see a patient with abdominal distension and a suspicion of volvulus, you must see the patient urgently.
- The goals for sigmoid volvulus include early diagnosis and endoscopic decompression as a temporizing measure until definite surgical management can be performed.
  - ¤ If the diagnosis is not clear from plain films, consider CT scan, water-soluble contrast enema, or consider proceeding to flexible sigmoidoscopy for diagnosis and decompression.
  - ¤ Endoscopic decompression for a sigmoid volvulus has a success rate of up to 80%, so it should be pursued unless there are peritoneal signs or concerns for perforation or gangrenous bowel.
  - ¤ Indications for surgical management: If there are signs of peritonitis on exam or perforation on imaging.
  - ¤ The success rate of endoscopic decompression for cecal volvulus and transverse colon volvulus is much lower and, thus, is usually surgically managed.

---

*The medicine team calls you for a consult on a 67-year-old man who was admitted 4 days prior after his daughter noted he had a productive cough, fever, and shortness of breath at home. He was diagnosed with a left lower-lobe pneumonia, has improved on IV antibiotics, and remains afebrile. Since admission, he has developed abdominal distension, obstipation, and pain associated with nausea and vomiting. The medicine team ordered an abdominal x-ray, which demonstrated a massively dilated colon with a cecal diameter of 10 cm. After discussion with a radiologist, they ordered additional imaging to evaluate for a possible obstruction. The CT scan demonstrated a diffusely dilated colon without obstruction, volvulus, or perforation. There is air noted in all segments of the colon. The medicine team is concerned for Ogilvie's syndrome and asks you what to do next. So far, they have initiated conservative measures, making the patient NPO, starting IV fluids, placing an NG tube, and sending off labs to check for electrolyte abnormalities.*

## PSEUDO-OBSTRUCTION

- Defined as acute colonic dilation, sometimes massive, without mechanical obstruction. Based on clinical presentation, pseudo-obstruction syndromes can be divided into chronic and acute forms.
  - o Acute colonic pseudo-obstruction (ACPO), also known as Ogilvie's syndrome, is an acute, severe colonic ileus.
    - Mechanical obstruction and toxic megacolon (acute toxic colitis) should be excluded before making a diagnosis of ACPO. Potential causes of toxic megacolon include the following: inflammatory bowel disease, infection (*Clostridium difficile*), ischemia, or radiation.
    - Spontaneous perforation ranges from 3% to 15%, with a high mortality rate if this occurs (at least 50%). Cecal diameter of more than 12 cm or duration of more than 6 days increases rate of complications.[4]
    - Predisposing factors include postsurgical patients, or those with underlying comorbidities such as advanced age, sepsis, hypothyroidism, electrolyte disturbances, renal insufficiency, medications, neurological disorders, or cardiac and respiratory disorders.

- Other populations at risk include spinal cord injury patients, severe burn patients, or those with retroperitoneal trauma.
- Infectious causes of ACPO include herpes simplex, varicella zoster, Epstein-Barr virus, and cytomegalovirus.[4]
  - Chronic intestinal pseudo-obstruction and chronic idiopathic intestinal pseudo-obstructions are motility disorders. The underlying etiologies, diagnostic challenges, and treatments are chronic in nature and are beyond the scope of this chapter.

## WHAT ARE YOUR NEXT STEPS?

- Your initial questions for the primary team should include the following:
  - When did the team first note onset of abdominal distension and obstructive symptoms?
  - Are there concerning abdominal exam findings, such as peritoneal signs? If so, surgery should be called emergently to evaluate the patient.
  - How dilated is the colon on imaging, and are there signs of ischemia and/or perforation?
- General initial recommendations to the primary team include the following:
  - Reverse and treat any electrolyte disturbances. Obtain a basic metabolic panel, magnesium, calcium, phosphorus, and CBC with differential. Consider checking thyroid function if clinically indicated.
  - Does the patient have underlying infection or sepsis? An appropriate work-up should be performed.
  - Patient should be NPO, receive IV fluids for maintaining euvolemic volume status, and have adequate IV access.

**Table 5-1.**

## PREDISPOSING CONDITIONS ASSOCIATED WITH ACUTE COLONIC PSEUDO-OBSTRUCTION
(based on a review of 400 cases)

- Trauma (nonoperative)
- Infection (pneumonia, sepsis most common)
- Cardiac (myocardial infarction, heart failure)
- Obstetric/gynecologic surgery
- Abdominal/pelvic surgery
- Neurologic (Parkinson's disease, spinal chord injury, multiple sclerosis, Alzheimer's disease)
- Orthopedic surgery
- Miscellaneous medical conditions (metabolic, cancer, respiratory failure, renal failure)
- Miscellaneous surgical conditions (urologic, thoracic, neurosurgery)

Associated conditions of approximately 400 patients.[5] Some patients had more than one associated condition.

- Making a diagnosis of ACPO
  - Review the patient's chart for additional history to help elicit predisposing risk factors for ACPO (Table 5-1).
    - While all postoperative patients are at risk for ACPO, it is most commonly seen in patients who have undergone orthopedic surgeries, abdominal surgeries, and cardiothoracic/vascular surgeries. In a single-center study, risk of ACPO was highest in patients who had undergone kidney or liver transplants and hip replacements.
    - Identify treatable medical causes of ACPO, including electrolyte disturbances, underlying infections, or medications.

- o Physical exam will help assess severity and/or potential contraindications to neostigmine.
  - Vital sign abnormalities such as tachycardia, hypotension, or fevers. Additionally, underlying bradycardia should be noted.
  - Respiratory exam to assess for wheezing, copious secretions, or labored breathing.
  - Abdominal exam to assess for pain on palpation, degree of distension, and peritoneal signs. Also, examine the abdomen for surgical scars; those with a history of colon cancer or partial colonic resection were excluded from receiving neostigmine.[6]
- Laboratory studies
  - o CBC with differential, basic metabolic panel, magnesium, phosphorus, calcium.
  - o *C. difficile* infection should be ruled out.
- Review imaging
  - o Abdominal x-ray: Dilated colon with air present in all colonic segments. Mechanical obstruction must be excluded. If mechanical obstruction or toxic megacolon cannot be excluded, consider additional imaging.
  - o Widest diameter of colonic dilation should be documented, but understand that colonic diameter alone does not determine risk of perforation. Acuity of onset and duration of dilation are other factors.
    - More than 12 cm cecal diameter and more than 9 cm for the transverse colon are the thresholds quoted for increased risk of perforation.
  - o CT is helpful to exclude mechanical obstruction and evaluate for other potential etiologies, such as colitis or toxic megacolon. Contrast enemas can also be considered to exclude obstruction.

## Management Recommendations for Acute Colonic Pseudo-Obstruction

- Conservative measures can be considered for 24 to 48 hours in patients without severe colonic distension or pain (Figure 5-3).
- Seventy-seven percent of patients in a retrospective review responded to conservative therapy with a mean duration of 4 days. Postoperative patients and those receiving narcotics tended to respond less to conservative therapy, but this was not statistically significant.
  - Bowel rest, NG tube decompression, volume and electrolyte repletion.
  - Medications to avoid: Any agents that may decrease GI motility including opiates, calcium-channel blockers, and anticholinergics.
  - Rectal tube decompression should be considered.
  - Mobilize patient if not contraindicated. Patient should alternate between left lateral decubitus and right lateral decubitus every hour. Other positioning measures include a "fetal position" with knees to chest or prone position with hips elevated on a pillow.
  - Serial abdominal exams to monitor for progressive abdominal distension or peritoneal signs. Consider serial abdominal plain films daily. Order a STAT supine and upright abdominal plain film if there is concern for perforation on physical exam.
  - Pharmacologic therapy can be considered if conservative measures fail, cecal diameter is more than 12 cm or duration of distension is more than 6 days, and no contraindications for neostigmine are present.
    - Neostigmine 2 mg IV over 3 to 5 minutes has been proven effective in a small, double-blinded randomized placebo-controlled trial.[6]

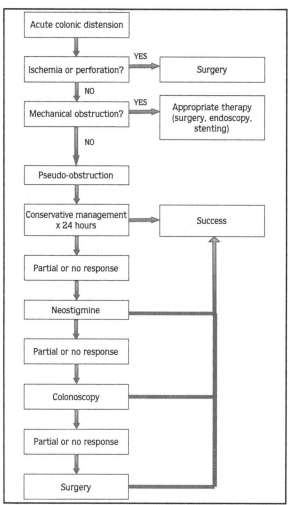

**Figure 5-3.** Algorithm for management of acute colonic pseudo-obstruction. (Adapted from Harrison ME, Anderson MA, Appalaneni V, et al. The role of endoscopy in the management of patients with known and suspected colonic obstruction and pseudo-obstruction. *Gastrointest Endosc.* 2010;71:669-679.)

Immediate clinical response was defined as evacuation of flatus or stool and decrease in abdominal distension within 30 minutes of infusion. Median response time was 4 minutes. Ninety-one percent of patients randomized to neostigmine had an immediate response, whereas none of the patients with placebo did. Twenty-seven percent of patients who received neostigmine required additional therapy (either colonic decompression or additional dose of neostigmine).

- Exclusion criteria: Suspected ischemia or perforation, pregnancy, active bronchospasm, baseline heart rate less than 60 beats per minute, cisapride or metoclopramide 24 hours before evaluation, active GI bleeding, history of colon cancer or partial colonic resection, and creatinine more than 3 mg/dL.

- Contraindications include hypersensitivity to neostigmine or bromides and GI or genitourinary obstruction. Relative contraindications include asthma; cardiac arrhythmias; recent myocardial infarction; or history of peptic ulcer disease, hyperthyroidism, or seizures.[7]

- Neostigmine may enhance the bradycardic effect of certain beta-blockers, cholinergic agonists, systemic corticosteroids, neuromuscular blocking agents, or succinylcholine. Adjust dose for renal insufficiency.

- Atropine should be at the bedside in case of symptomatic bradycardia; patients should be on continuous electrocardiographic monitoring and should be kept supine 60 minutes after the injection.

- Clinical pearl: The rationale for neostigmine treatment is that the pathophysiology of ACPO is thought to be related to dysregulation of sympathetic stimuli, which normally decreases colonic motility, and parasympathetic stimuli, which normally increases colonic motility to the colon. Neostigmine, an acetylcholinesterase inhibitor, is thought to cause rapid colonic decompression by increasing parasympathetic stimuli via increased levels of acetylcholine.
    - Prior to treatment, it is helpful to inform the primary team and nursing staff to monitor for parasympathetic symptoms such as excess salivation, miosis, sweating, hyperperistalsis (vomiting or diarrhea), bronchoconstriction, and bradycardia. Neostigmine can also induce seizures, hypotension, and asystole.
- Can a second dose of neostigmine be given if the first dose fails? There is insufficient evidence to recommend for or against this, so use your clinical judgment for each patient.
- If treatment with neostigmine results in colonic decompression, consider recommending a bowel regimen to prevent constipation and improve colonic motility.
    - Examples include low-volume cathartic agents such as lactulose, low-dose polyethylene glycol, or bisacodyl suppositories.
- Endoscopic decompression should be considered for patients who have a contraindication for neostigmine, have failed neostigmine, and who do not have evidence of obstruction or perforation on imaging and/or peritoneal signs on abdominal exam.
    - Successful endoscopic decompression has been reported in retrospective studies. There are no trials directly comparing neostigmine to endoscopic therapy. Overall clinical success of colonic decompression was 88%. Eighteen percent required multiple (2 to 4) decompressions. Perforation occurred in 2%.[8]

○ If sedation is required, benzodiazepines alone should suffice. Efforts should be made to avoid narcotics, which decrease colonic motility and may exacerbate ACPO.

○ Minimal air should be insufflated with suctioning of as much gas and stool as possible to minimize risk of perforation. Decompression is generally sufficient if the endoscope reaches the hepatic flexure.

○ Decompression tubes can be placed in the right colon with the aid of a guidewire and fluoroscopic guidance. Once placed, it should be drained to gravity and flushed every 4 hours to prevent clogging.

- Surgical options include cecostomy or colectomy, but they have a higher morbidity and mortality rate (30% and 6%, respectively) compared with pharmacologic and endoscopic options. It is generally reserved for those patients who have complications from ACPO, such as perforation, or who have failed pharmacologic and endoscopic efforts.

---

### Key Points to Acute Colonic Pseudo-Obstruction

- Important differential causes to exclude include mechanical obstruction and toxic megacolon. Colonic diameter alone does not determine risk of perforation. Acuity of onset and duration of dilation are other factors.
- For conservative management, reversible or treatable risk factors for ACPO should be identified and treated, along with supportive care.
- Neostigmine 2 mg IV given over 3 to 5 minutes should yield a rapid response in the majority of patients. After first excluding contraindications to neostigmine, we have the patient monitored on telemetry while it is being administered. Atropine should be easily

(*continued*)

---

### Key Points to Acute Colonic Pseudo-Obstruction (continued)

accessible. The most common side effect is transient abdominal cramping. Important side effects include symptomatic bradycardia and bronchospasm. A repeat dose can be considered if there is no response or a partial response.

- Colonic decompression has a good clinical success rate and should be considered in those who have a contraindication to neostigmine or who have failed neostigmine in the absence of peritoneal signs or perforation.
- Consider surgical options for patients in whom pharmacologic or endoscopic measures have failed or who have signs of perforation or peritoneal signs.

# REFERENCES

1. Jones DJ. ABC of colorectal disease. Large bowel volvulus. *BMJ.* 1992;305(6849):358-360.
2. Safioleas M, Chatziconstantinou C, Felekouras E, et al. Clinical considerations and therapeutic strategy for sigmoid volvulus in the elderly: a study of 33 cases. *World J Gastroenterol.* 2007;13(6):921-924.
3. Grossmann EM, Longo WE, Stratton MD, Virgo KS, Johnson FE. Sigmoid volvulus in Department of Veterans Affairs Medical Centers. *Dis Colon Rectum.* 2000;43:414-418.
4. Saunders MD. Acute colonic pseudo-obstruction. *Best Practice Res Clin Gastroenterol.* 2007;21(4):671-687.
5. Vanek VW, Al-Salti M. Acute colonic pseudo-obstruction of the colon (Ogilvie's syndrome). An analysis of 400 cases. *Dis Colon Rectum.* 1986;29:203-210.
6. Ponec RJ, Saunders MD, Kimmey MB. Neostigmine for the treatment of acute colonic pseudo-obstruction. *N Engl J Med.* 1999;341(3):137-141.
7. Loftus CG, Harewood GC, Baron TH. Assessment of predictors of response to neostigmine for acute colonic pseudo-obstruction. *Am J Gastroenterol.* 2002;97(12):3118-3122.
8. Geller A, Petersen BT, Gostout CJ. Endoscopic decompression for acute colonic pseudo-obstruction. *Gastrointest Endosc.* 1996;44(2):144-150.

# 6

# Fulminant Colitis

*Sharmeel K. Wasan, MD*
*Francis A. Farraye, MD, MSc*

You receive the following call from the emergency department (ED):

> *We have a 32-year-old woman with a history of ulcerative colitis (UC) who presents to the ED with bloody diarrhea and fever for the past 2 days. She does not look well, has a pulse of 110 and a blood pressure (BP) of 110/60. Should we start steroids?*

- Initial response
  - Try to determine how "sick" the patient is.
    - Clinical criteria for an acute attack of severe UC consists of the following features:
      - Diarrhea.
      - The presence of one or more of the following signs: Obvious blood in the stool, fever, pulse >90, hemoglobin <10.5 g/L, and erythrocyte sedimentation rate (ESR) >30 mm/h2.[1]
- About 10% to 15% of UC patients will develop a severe episode of colitis requiring hospitalization.
- About 1% to 2% will develop fulminant colitis.

Lowe RC, Farraye FA.
*GI Emergencies: A Quick Reference Guide* (pp 91-106).
© 2012 Taylor & Francis Group

- Before the use of steroids, the mortality for severe UC was 25% to 60%. Mortality now remains at 1% to 2% for fulminant colitis patients.[2]

*You proceed into the hospital. What questions should you ask the patient to complete the history?*

- Find out more about her UC.
  - What was the extent of her disease in the past?
    - When was her last colonoscopy and how much of her colon was involved?
    - Has she ever had an evaluation of her small intestine to exclude the possibility of Crohn's disease (CD)?
      - Determining UC versus CD is important and will affect the surgical approach should surgery become necessary. UC patients are candidates for an ileal pouch-anal anastomosis (IPAA) while the procedure is not recommended for CD patients.
  - What medications was she taking?
    - Is the patient immunocompromised from any of the medications (ie, steroids, immunomodulators, or biologics)?
      - If the patient is immunocompromised, this may put her at risk for infection.
    - Has she ever needed steroids in the past? How many times?
      - The need for corticosteroids in UC is associated with a more aggressive disease pattern and a worse prognosis.
  - Ask about travel.
  - Ask about recent antibiotic use.
  - Ask if she was taking nonsteroidal anti-inflammatory drugs.

*On further history, you determine that the patient was first diagnosed with left-sided UC when she was 20 years old. Since her diagnosis, she has required 3 courses of oral steroids. She normally takes a*

*5-aminosalicylic acid (5-ASA) agent, but she for-
got to take her medications during a business trip
2 weeks ago. As her symptoms were worsening, she
started 40 mg of prednisone on her own 2 days ago.*

*On physical examination, you find that the patient
remains tachycardic despite 2 L normal saline given
in the emergency room. Her abdomen is soft and
nondistended but with diffuse tenderness to palpation, most prominent in the left lower quadrant.
There is no rebound or guarding.*

*Initial laboratory analysis reveals WBC 13, Hct 28,
MCV 80, Plts 530 K. Chemistry and liver function
panels are remarkable only for an albumin of 3.4.*

- The patient meets criteria for severe UC (Table 6-1).
- However, before the diagnosis can be confirmed, it
  is very important to rule out other etiologies for her
  symptoms.
  - Initial tests that should be obtained
    - Check for *Clostridium difficile* toxin.
      - Superimposed *C. difficile* infection is very
        common in the inflammatory bowel dis-
        ease (IBD) patient. In fact, patients with *C.
        difficile* infection and IBD are nearly 6 times
        more likely to undergo bowel surgery than
        IBD patients without *C. difficile*.[3,4]
      - It is important to check at least 3 stool sam-
        ples to increase the sensitivity of the test.
      - If your patient tests positive for *C. difficile*,
        it is reasonable to begin therapy with oral
        vancomycin or to make an early switch
        to oral vancomycin from metronidazole
        if the patient has not improved within
        48 hours. The newest guidelines recom-
        mend vancomycin for patients with se-
        vere colitis.
    - Check stool cultures for enteric pathogens
      (Salmonella, Shigella, etc).
    - Check stool for ova and parasites.
    - Kidney, ureter, and bladder (KUB) x-ray.

Table 6-1.

## COLITIS ACTIVITY ASSESSMENT

|  | MILD | MODERATE | SEVERE | FULMINANT |
|---|---|---|---|---|
| Stools (#/day) | <4 | >4 | >6 | >10 |
| Blood in stool | Intermittent | Intermittent | Frequent | Continuous |
| Temp (°C) | Normal | Normal | >37.5 | >37.5 |
| Pulse | Normal | Normal | >90 | >90 |
| Hemoglobin | Normal | Normal | <75% of normal | Transfusion required |
| ESR | <30 | <30 | >30 | >30 |
| Radiographic | Normal | Normal | Thumb printing | Dilated colon |
| ABD Exam | Normal | Normal | Tender, no rebound | Distended, ↓ BS, +/- rebound |

Adapted from Kornbluth A, Sachar DB, Practice Parameters Committee of the American College of Gastroenterology. Ulcerative colitis practice guidelines in adults. *Am J Gastroenterol.* 2010;105(3):501-523.

- Surgical consult.
  - Working with a surgeon early in the clinical course will allow for the best outcome and ideally prevent the need for emergent colectomy.
  - Short-term mortality after surgery for UC was found to be higher in those who had emergency surgery than those who underwent elective surgery.[5]

*You determine that the patient has severe UC based on her history and physical exam as well as the negative stool studies. What next?*

- Stop 5-ASA agents in most cases of patients with severe colitis.
  - Little additional benefit from 5-ASA agents with steroids.
  - Rare idiosyncratic reaction in which 5-ASA agents are associated with an exacerbation of colitis.
- No benefit seen from bowel rest. Therefore, no reason to make the patient NPO (nothing by mouth).
  - In patients with fulminant colitis, patients should be NPO given the possibility of emergency surgery and associated nausea and vomiting.
    - Consider intravenous (IV) nutrition in the severely malnourished patient.
- Hold off on empiric use of antibiotics in all patients. Although they are often used, randomized controlled trials have shown no benefit.
- Check daily KUB.
- Avoid narcotics and anticholinergic agents.
- Begin treatment of IV corticosteroids (Figure 6-1).
  - No need to overdose corticosteroids—no benefit seen with doses higher than 60 mg of prednisone.[6]
    - Hydrocortisone 100 mg IV q8 hour.
    - Methylprednisolone sodium succinate (Solu-Medrol) 20 mg IV q8 hour.
  - Continuous infusion of IV corticosteroids is not more efficacious than bolus dosing.[7]
  - Re-assess regularly (once to twice daily) in the next 3 to 5 days.
    - If no response to corticosteroids, then need to consider next step.
    - Consider transfer to a hospital with an IBD center if no response.
    - Expect that about 60% of patients will be symptom-free at 5 days, 15% will have a significant improvement, and 25% of patients will end up needing infliximab, cyclosporine, or surgery.[8]

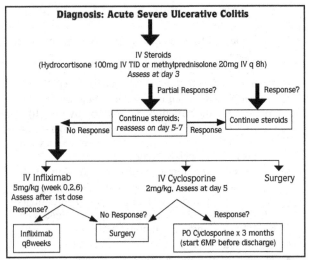

**Figure 6-1.** Treatment algorithm for acute severe UC. (Adapted from Hart AL, Ng SC. Review article: the optimal medical management of acute severe ulcerative colitis. *Aliment Pharmacol Ther.* 2010;32(5):615-627.)

*The patient is placed on IV corticosteroids. On day 3, she states that she is feeling about the same. She continues to have mild diffuse tenderness to palpation on physical examination, and her KUB is unremarkable. She continues to complain of 10 bloody bowel movements a day. She has met with the surgical team upon your request, but continues to be very resistant to the idea of surgery.*

- Because she is not responding to IV steroids, plan for an unprepared flexible sigmoidoscopy to assess disease severity of UC and to obtain mucosal biopsies to rule out cytomegalovirus (CMV).[9,10]
    - Avoid total colonoscopy and ileoscopy because the air insufflation can induce a toxic megacolon.

- ○ Findings on biopsy of CMV:
  - ▪ Viral intranuclear inclusions (that can be confirmed by immunohistochemistry).
  - ▪ Other nonspecific changes: Focal cryptitis, increased epithelial cell apoptosis.
- ○ If biopsies demonstrate CMV, then treatment with ganciclovir or foscarnet has been shown to have good response, and patients are often able to quickly taper off steroids.
- ○ Endoscopy findings can also assist in prognostication.
  - ▪ Deep ulcerations predict a poor response to medical therapy.[11]

*Flexible sigmoidoscopy demonstrates severe UC with deep ulcerations and friable mucosa. Biopsies are taken, and there is no evidence of viral inclusion bodies to indicate CMV infection. She is presented with the following options: cyclosporine, infliximab, or surgery (see Figure 6-1).*

## MEDICAL MANAGEMENT: CYCLOSPORINE

- Use of cyclosporine has been shown to decrease the need for short-term colectomy.[12]
  - ○ Overall, in about 60% to 80% of patients, cyclosporine prevents colectomy in the short-term, with about 50% avoiding colectomy in the long-term.[13]
- Transitioning to maintenance therapy with 6-mercaptopurine (6-MP) or azathioprine (AZA) has been shown to decrease long-term need for colectomy.[14]
- Predictive factors for poor response to cyclosporine and need for colectomy[15]:
  - ○ Temperature >37.5°C, heart rate >90, C-reactive protein (CRP) >45 mg/L.
  - ○ Presence of severe endoscopic lesions.

- Things to do before starting cyclosporine:
    - Obtain the following baseline studies:
        - Creatinine clearance (>30% reduction in the glomerular filtration rate is a contraindication to therapy).
        - Cholesterol (<120 mg/dL is a contraindication to therapy).
        - Magnesium (must be maintained >1.5 mg/dL).
        - TPMT enzyme activity in anticipation of starting 6-MP/AZA upon discharge.
    - Rule out active infection.
- Therapy protocol
    - Dose of IV cyclosporine: 2 mg/kg/day.
    - Continue IV steroids.
    - Prophylactic trimethoprim/sulfamethoxazole (TMP-SMZ).
- Monitoring
    - Cyclosporine levels every day; goal 200 to 300 ng/mL.
    - Follow daily labs, especially for Cr, K, Mg, and liver function tests.
    - Daily serum cholesterol (total parenteral nutrition with lipids if persistently low to prevent seizures).
    - Daily monitoring for paresthesias.
    - Vitals; monitor for hypertension.
- If patient responds to cyclosporine:
    - Transition to oral cyclosporine (give 2 times the IV dose split twice daily).
    - Change to oral prednisone with slow taper.
    - Continue TMP-SMZ.
    - Add 6-MP/AZA prior to discharge from the hospital.
    - Discontinue cyclosporine therapy after 3 to 6 months.
    - Remember to monitor weekly cyclosporine levels with a goal of 150 to 300 ng/mL, complete blood count, electrolytes.

# MEDICAL MANAGEMENT: INFLIXIMAB

- What is the evidence behind the use of infliximab?
  - In a trial of 45 inpatients with moderate to severe UC not responding to 3 to 7 days of IV corticosteroids, a single dose of infliximab at 5 mg/kg prevented colectomy in 71% of patients. In contrast, 67% of patients in the placebo group underwent colectomy.[16]
  - The efficacy of infliximab for the induction and maintenance of remission in outpatients with moderate to severe UC was evaluated in 2 randomized, double-blind, placebo-controlled trials (the Active Ulcerative Trials 1 and 2).[17]
  - Infliximab induces and maintains clinical response, clinical remission, and mucosal healing.
    - Infliximab enables patients with active UC to discontinue corticosteroids and achieve remission.
  - In a review of 34 studies of 896 patients with moderate to severe UC, remission was achieved in 40% of infliximab patients at 9 months follow-up.[18]
- Predictors of poor response to infliximab[19,20]:
  - Peripheral antineutrophil cytoplasmic antibodies positive and/or anti-*Saccharomyces cerevisiae* antibodies-negative serotype.
  - Older age.
  - Disease duration of less than 3 years.
  - Bowel frequency more than 6 times a day on admission.
  - Prior hospitalization in the past 3 months for UC.
  - Low serum albumin on day of admission and day 3 of IV steroids.
- Does infliximab lead to postoperative complications in UC?
  - Although controversial, recent studies suggest that there is no difference in complication rates

after surgery between patients who received infliximab within 12 weeks of surgery and those who did not.[21]

- Things to do before starting infliximab:
  - Check for tuberculosis (PPD; given concern for anergy issues, check chest x-ray).
  - Check HBsAg.
  - Rule out superimposed CMV, *C. difficile*.
- Therapy protocol:
  - Induction dosing of infliximab.
    - 5 mg/kg—round to the closest 100 mg.
    - Give three doses at 0, 2, and 6 weeks.
  - Maintenance dosing of infliximab every 8 weeks.

*Cyclosporine has failed. Should I now try infliximab?*
*Infliximab has failed. Should I now try cyclosporine?*

- Switching from cyclosporine to infliximab or vice versa has significant risks.
  - In a retrospective chart review of 19 patients who failed cyclosporine and then were treated with infliximab (n = 10) or who failed infliximab first and then were treated with cyclosporine (n = 6) within 4 weeks of discontinuing the initial drug, 3 serious adverse events were noted (herpetic esophagitis, jaundice, and death).[22]
  - Thus, most experts have recommended not trying a second agent after the patient fails to respond to the initial drug due to concern of increased risk of infection and postoperative complications with preoperative exposures to both agents.

# SURGERY

- Predictors of colectomy
  - Stool frequency of >8/day on day 3 or a CRP >45 mg/L in patients still passing 3 to 8 stools per day resulted in an 85% colectomy rate.[23]

- Complications of surgery: IPAA.[24-26]
  - Patients considered for surgery should be advised about the risks and benefits of the surgery within their specific clinical setting.
  - The IPAA has become the operation of choice for patients with UC.
  - Risk of mortality of <0.5%.
  - Decrease in female fertility (infertility rate of 39% to 82%).
  - Other risks of IPAA include the following:
    - Pouchitis (10% to 60%).
    - Small bowel obstruction (20%).
    - CD of the pouch (2.7% to 13%).
    - Pouch-vaginal fistula (4%).
- Remember, if surgery is delayed, there is a higher risk of morbidity and mortality.

*Despite your recommendation, the patient refuses all of the above options after consulting with a family friend who is also a physician who advises her to continue to try 2 more days of steroids. Unfortunately, on day 7 of IV steroids, she begins to look worse. She is having 8 bloody bowel movements a day. On physical exam, she has a temperature of 101.5°F, BP of 85/60, and heart rate of 120. She now has diffuse abdominal tenderness with distention. Laboratory work reveals a WBC 16, Hct 24, Plts 670. Albumin is now 2.4. A KUB is performed and reveals marked dilation of the transverse colon to 10 cm. A repeat C. difficile is again negative.*

- Based on the above clinical, laboratory, and imaging data, the patient now meets criteria for toxic megacolon, a life-threatening complication of fulminant colitis. The diagnosis of toxic megacolon is based on clinical information and plain x-rays of the abdomen.
  - The typical clinical presentation includes diarrhea, bloody diarrhea, constipation, obstipation,

abdominal pain, tenderness and distention, and decreased bowel sounds.

o Findings on a CT scan (if performed) would demonstrate colonic dilation, diffuse colonic wall thickening, submucosal edema, pericolonic stranding, perforations, and abscesses.

o Clinical criteria as described by Jalan et al[27] should include any 3 of the following 4 points:

1. Fever >101.5°F (38.6°C).
2. Heart rate >120 beats/min.
3. White blood cell count >10.5.
4. Anemia.

- In addition, patients should also have one of the following: dehydration, mental status changes, electrolyte disturbances, or hypotension.

o Other causes of toxic megacolon include the following[28]:

- Ischemia
- Infectious etiologies (C. difficile, Salmonella, Shigella, Yersinia, Campylobacter, Cryptosporidium, Entameba, CMV)
- Malignancy (such as Kaposi's sarcoma)

o Management of toxic megacolon:

- General: IV support, correct electrolyte abnormalities, complete bowel rest, stop all anticholinergic agents and narcotics, rule out infectious etiologies.
- Decompression: Rectal tube, nasogastric tube, repositioning maneuvers.
- Medical care: Specific treatment for infections, broad-spectrum antibiotics, IV corticosteroids.
- Radiology: Frequent assessment with plain films.
- Early surgical consultation.

- Surgical intervention[29] in patients with failed medical therapy, progressive toxicity or dilation, or signs of perforation.
  - Surgical procedure of choice in urgent situations: Turnbull-Blowhole operation with subsequent elective colectomy or subtotal colectomy and ileostomy.
  - Surgical procedure in more elective situations: Total colectomy and ileostomy.
- The development of toxic megacolon is associated with high mortality rates, with significantly higher rates in patients requiring emergency surgery for perforation.
  - Interestingly, mortality does not seem to be related to the extent of the underlying disease (ie, no difference in pancolitis versus limited colitis).
  - Fecal soilage and sepsis are often the cause of postoperative mortality.

*Based on the criteria discussed above, a diagnosis of toxic megacolon is made, and the patient is taken to the operating room. She undergoes a subtotal colectomy and ileostomy. Pathology confirms the diagnosis of severe UC. The patient recovered rapidly after the surgery and was discharged home on postoperative day 5 with a follow-up plan for proctectomy and IPAA.*

---

## Key Points

- The number of bowel movements, presence of blood in the stool, temperature, pulse, hemoglobin, ESR, abdominal exam, and radiographic findings are important criteria to help characterize the severity of a UC flare.
- Before concluding that the patient has a flare of severe UC, it is important to rule out other infectious etiologies, particularly *C. difficile* and CMV.

*(continued)*

### Key Points (continued)

- Patients with IBD are particularly susceptible to *C. difficile* infections.
- Performing an early flexible sigmoidoscopy is important to help confirm the diagnosis of UC and rule out CMV by biopsies.
- For confirmed severe UC, a 3-day trial of IV corticosteroids is the recommended first step.
  - For those patients who respond to IV steroids, switch to PO steroids with a plan for a slow taper and consider starting 6-MP/AZA.
  - For those patients who do not respond to IV steroids in the first 3 to 5 days, the next step would be to proceed with infliximab, cyclosporine, or surgery depending on the particular patient.
- Infliximab is easy to use and induces and maintains clinical response, clinical remission, and mucosal healing.
- IV cyclosporine is effective, but requires close monitoring of cholesterol, electrolytes, renal function, and blood pressure. If the patient responds to cyclosporine therapy, 6-MP/AZA should be started prior to hospital discharge.
- One randomized controlled study in hospitalized steroid refractory UC patients showed equal efficacy of cyclosporine and infliximab.
- It is not recommended to try infliximab after cyclosporine failure or vice versa due to concern for increased infectious complications.
- It is important not to delay surgery when indicated.
- Toxic megacolon is a life-threatening complication of fulminant colitis.

## REFERENCES

1. Truelove SC, Witts LJ. Cortisone in ulcerative colitis; final report on a therapeutic trial. *Br Med J.* 1955;2(4947):1041-1048.
2. Truelove SC, Jewell DP. Intensive intravenous regimen for severe attacks of ulcerative colitis. *Lancet.* 1974;1(7866):1067-1070.
3. Ananthakrishnan AN, McGinley EL, Binion DG. Excess hospitalization burden associated with *Clostridium difficile* in patients with inflammatory bowel disease. *Gut.* 2008;57(2):205-210.

4. Jodorkovsky D, Young Y, Abreu MT. Clinical outcomes of patients with ulcerative colitis and co-existing *Clostridium difficile* infection. *Dig Dis Sci.* 2010;55(2):415-420.

5. Kaplan GG, McCarthy EP, Ayanian JZ, Korzenik J, Hodin R, Sands BE. Impact of hospital volume on postoperative morbidity and mortality following a colectomy for ulcerative colitis. *Gastroenterology.* 2008;134(3):680-687.

6. Rosenberg W, Ireland A, Jewell DP. High-dose methylprednisolone in the treatment of active ulcerative colitis. *J Clin Gastroenterol.* 1990;12(1):40-41.

7. Bossa F, Fiorella S, Caruso N, et al. Continuous infusion versus bolus administration of steroids in severe attacks of ulcerative colitis: a randomized, double-blind trial. *Am J Gastroenterol.* 2007;102(3):601-608.

8. Turner D, Walsh CM, Steinhart AH, Griffiths AM. Response to corticosteroids in severe ulcerative colitis: a systematic review of the literature and a meta-regression. *Clin Gastroenterol Hepatol.* 2007;5(1):103-110.

9. Alemayehu G, Jarnerot G. Colonoscopy during an attack of severe ulcerative colitis is a safe procedure and of great value in clinical decision making. *Am J Gastroenterol.* 1991;86(2):187-190.

10. Diepersloot RJ, Kroes AC, Visser W, Jiwa NM, Rothbarth PH. Acute ulcerative proctocolitis associated with primary cytomegalovirus infection. *Arch Intern Med.* 1990;150(8):1749-1751.

11. Carbonnel F, Gargouri D, Lemann M, et al. Predictive factors of outcome of intensive intravenous treatment for attacks of ulcerative colitis. *Aliment Pharmacol Ther.* 2000;14(3):273-279.

12. Lichtiger S, Present DH, Kornbluth A, et al. Cyclosporine in severe ulcerative colitis refractory to steroid therapy. *N Engl J Med.* 1994;330(26):1841-1845.

13. Arts J, D'Haens G, Zeegers M, et al. Long-term outcome of treatment with intravenous cyclosporin in patients with severe ulcerative colitis. *Inflamm Bowel Dis.* 2004;10(2):73-78.

14. Cohen RD, Stein R, Hanauer SB. Intravenous cyclosporin in ulcerative colitis: a five-year experience. *Am J Gastroenterol.* 1999;94(6):1587-1592.

15. Cacheux W, Seksik P, Lemann M, et al. Predictive factors of response to cyclosporine in steroid-refractory ulcerative colitis. *Am J Gastroenterol.* 2008;103(3):637-642.

16. Jarnerot G, Hertervig E, Friis-Liby I, et al. Infliximab as rescue therapy in severe to moderately severe ulcerative colitis: a randomized, placebo-controlled study. *Gastroenterology.* 2005;128(7):1805-1811.

17. Rutgeerts P, Sandborn WJ, Feagan BG, et al. Infliximab for induction and maintenance therapy for ulcerative colitis. *N Engl J Med.* 2005;353(23):2462-2476.

18. Gisbert JP, Gonzalez-Lama Y, Mate J. Systematic review: Infliximab therapy in ulcerative colitis. *Aliment Pharmacol Ther.* 2007;25(1):19-37.

19. Ferrante M, Vermeire S, Katsanos KH, et al. Predictors of early response to infliximab in patients with ulcerative colitis. *Inflamm Bowel Dis.* 2007;13(2):123-128.

20. Lees CW, Heys D, Ho GT, et al. A retrospective analysis of the efficacy and safety of infliximab as rescue therapy in acute severe ulcerative colitis. *Aliment Pharmacol Ther.* 2007;26(3):411-419.

21. Kunitake H, Hodin R, Shellito PC, Sands BE, Korzenik J, Bordeianou L. Perioperative treatment with infliximab in patients with Crohn's disease and ulcerative colitis is not associated with an increased rate of postoperative complications. *J Gastrointest Surg.* 2008;12(10):1730-1736; discussion 1736-1737.

22. Maser EA, Deconda D, Lichtiger S, Ullman T, Present DH, Kornbluth A. Cyclosporine and infliximab as acute salvage therapies for each other, in severe steroid-refractory ulcerative colitis. *Gut.* 2007;132(S):1132.

23. Travis SP, Farrant JM, Ricketts C, et al. Predicting outcome in severe ulcerative colitis. *Gut.* 1996;38(6):905-910.

24. Becker JM. Surgical therapy for ulcerative colitis and Crohn's disease. *Gastroenterol Clin North Am.* 1999;28(2):371-390, viii-ix.

25. Johnson P, Richard C, Ravid A, et al. Female infertility after ileal pouch-anal anastomosis for ulcerative colitis. *Dis Colon Rectum.* 2004;47(7):1119-1126.

26. Pemberton JH, Kelly KA, Beart RW Jr, Dozois RR, Wolff BG, Ilstrup DM. Ileal pouch-anal anastomosis for chronic ulcerative colitis. Long-term results. *Ann Surg.* 1987;206(4):504-513.

27. Jalan KN, Sircus W, Card WI, et al. An experience of ulcerative colitis. I. Toxic dilation in 55 cases. *Gastroenterology.* 1969;57(1):68-82.

28. Gan, DI, Beck PL. A new look at toxic megacolon: an update and review of incidence, etiology, pathogenesis, and management. *Am J Gastroenterol.* 2003;98(11):2363-2371.

29. Turnbull RB Jr, Weakley FL, Hawk WA, Schofield P. Choice of operation for the toxic megacolon phase of nonspecific ulcerative colitis. *Surg Clin North Am.* 1970;50(5):1151-1169.

# 7

# Acute Pancreatitis

*Ivonne Ramirez, MD*
*David R. Lichtenstein, MD*

You receive the following call from the emergency department:

*A 48-year-old woman presents complaining of severe, sharp epigastric abdominal pain radiating to the back, which started about 4 hours prior to her presentation and is associated with bilious emesis. She recalls 2 prior episodes of abdominal pain over the past year but these have been located more toward her right upper quadrant, have not been as severe, have been associated with some nausea, and, although constant, the pain subsided both times without intervention after 2 or 3 hours.*

*Her past medical history includes hypertension and hyperlipidemia for which she is taking a beta-blocker, a statin, and an aspirin. She denies use of alcohol, tobacco, or illicit drugs.*

*Physical examination reveals a blood pressure of 150/95, heart rate of 114, $O_2$ saturation of 98% on room air, and temperature of 98.6°F. Weight is 165 lbs, and height is 5'4". In general, the patient*

Lowe RC, Farraye FA.
*GI Emergencies: A Quick Reference Guide* (pp 107-130).
© 2012 Taylor & Francis Group

*appears in some distress, preferring to sit up rather than lay supine. Her abdominal exam is notable for tenderness to palpation in the epigastric region with no guarding and no rebound tenderness. There is no hepatosplenomegaly.*

*Labs are notable for a WBC of 8,300/uL, amylase of 18,000 IU/L, and a lipase of 16,000 IU/L. Her alanine aminotransferase (ALT) is 170 IU/L and aspartate aminotransferase (AST) is 200 IU/L, alkaline phosphatase is 382 IU/L, and T bilirubin is 1.2 mg/dL. An abdominal ultrasound is performed, which is notable for gallstones but no gallbladder wall thickening or pericholecystic fluid. The maximal common bile duct (CBD) diameter is 9 mm. We have started intravenous (IV) fluids, and she is being admitted to a general medical floor.*

# CLINICAL PRESENTATION

The hallmark of acute pancreatitis (AP) is the acute onset of persistent pain, although in atypical cases, patients may present with unexplained multisystem organ failure or postoperative ileus. The spectrum of clinical manifestations and characteristics of the abdominal pain are described in Figure 7-1.

## ESTABLISH THE DIAGNOSIS OF ACUTE PANCREATITIS

Practice guidelines recommend establishing the diagnosis of AP within 48 hours of admission.[1-4] However, earlier diagnosis is preferred when possible in order to initiate appropriate treatment.

Demonstrate at least 2 of the following 3 features[1-3,5]:
- Characteristic abdominal pain.
  - o Acute onset of persistent upper abdominal pain often associated with nausea and vomiting.
  - o Pain is usually located in the epigastric and periumbilical regions and may radiate to the back, chest, flanks, and lower abdomen.

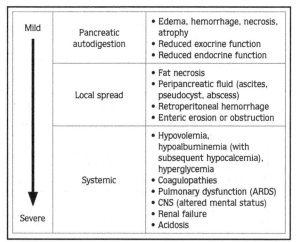

| Mild | Pancreatic autodigestion | • Edema, hemorrhage, necrosis, atrophy<br>• Reduced exocrine function<br>• Reduced endocrine function |
| | Local spread | • Fat necrosis<br>• Peripancreatic fluid (ascites, pseudocyst, abscess)<br>• Retroperitoneal hemorrhage<br>• Enteric erosion or obstruction |
| Severe | Systemic | • Hypovolemia, hypoalbuminemia (with subsequent hypocalcemia), hyperglycemia<br>• Coagulopathies<br>• Pulmonary dysfunction (ARDS)<br>• CNS (altered mental status)<br>• Renal failure<br>• Acidosis |

**Figure 7-1.** Clinical manifestations and complications of pancreatitis.

- o Patients are usually restless, and the supine position may increase the intensity of pain. Patients tend to bend forward (knee-chest position) in order to alleviate the pain.
- Serum amylase and/or lipase 3 or more times the upper limit of normal in patients without concomitant renal failure.
  - o Elevations in amylase or lipase levels less than 3 times the upper limit of normal have low specificity for AP and are consistent with but not diagnostic of AP.
  - o Serum pancreatic enzyme levels can be elevated in other processes being considered in the differential diagnosis, such as bowel perforation, intestinal obstruction, mesenteric ischemia, dissecting aortic aneurysm, and tubo-ovarian disease.
  - o Both amylase and lipase can be elevated in patients with renal insufficiency.

o If serum pancreatic enzymes remain elevated long-term, consider persistent inflammatory changes or development of a pancreatic duct leak or pseudocyst.

## AMYLASE

- Elevations may not occur or can be missed depending on the timing of measurement. This is a potential factor in mild cases, in acute superimposed on chronic pancreatitis, and in those with hypertriglyceridemia (can interfere with the assay).
- Amylase may be elevated in several nonpancreatic conditions, such as renal insufficiency and macroamylasemia.

## LIPASE

- May be preferable to amylase because it remains elevated longer (can remain elevated for more than 5 days).
- Considered slightly more specific than amylase. In contrast to amylase, it is normal in some nonpancreatic disorders including macroamylasemia, parotitis, and tubo-ovarian disease.
- Characteristic findings of AP on abdominal imaging:
  o Contrast-enhanced computed tomography (CECT) scanning is preferred for imaging the pancreas in suspected AP.
  o A CT scan on admission is only indicated when the diagnosis is in doubt.[2-4]
  o Characteristic findings on CT imaging include pancreatic enlargement, peripancreatic inflammatory changes, and peripancreatic fluid collections.
  o CT scan findings can also be useful for assessing the severity of pancreatitis and to identify complications of necrosis and peripancreatic fluid collections.

- o Early CT (within 72 hours of symptom onset) can underestimate the presence and amount of pancreatic necrosis.
- o The pancreas appears normal on CT scanning in 15% to 30% of mild cases.
- o Magnetic resonance imaging (MRI) with gadolinium enhancement is as accurate as CT in imaging the pancreas, determining severity of disease, and determining the degree of necrosis. However, MRI scanning is more difficult in critically ill patients and similarly carries a risk of contrast-induced renal failure.[2]

# INITIAL EVALUATION

## BEDSIDE ASSESSMENT

- Physical exam
  - o Assess patient's general appearance.
  - o Physical examination findings are variable and may include fever, hypotension, severe abdominal tenderness with focal peritoneal signs, respiratory distress, and abdominal distention.
    - Cullen's sign (periumbilical ecchymoses) or Grey Turner's sign (flank ecchymoses) can be seen in hemorrhagic pancreatitis. These physical exam findings are rare.
  - o Determine patient's volume status (orthostatics, urine output).

## DIAGNOSTIC TESTS TO PERFORM

1. On admission
   - Laboratory
     - o Amylase or lipase to help establish the diagnosis
       - There is no correlation between the severity of the pancreatitis and the level of elevation in amylase or lipase.

- No clear benefit has been shown in following amylase or lipase levels over time to gauge disease progression.
  - o Serum chemistry profile, blood urea nitrogen (BUN), complete blood count (CBC)
  - o $O_2$ saturation
  - o Triglyceride level, calcium level, liver profile (bilirubin, ALT, AST, alkaline phosphatase) to evaluate for etiologies
    - A 3-fold elevation in ALT has a 95% positive predictive value (PPV) for biliary pancreatitis.
- Imaging on admission[2-4]
  - o Transabdominal ultrasound is preferred to other imaging modalities for the initial evaluation to identify cholelithiasis. Ultrasound is insensitive for identifying choledocholithiasis but, when noted, is very specific.
  - o An initial CT scan is only recommended for evaluation when the presenting diagnosis is uncertain. Only perform after adequate fluid resuscitation to minimize the risk of contrast-induced nephrotoxicity. Also, recognize that early CT scanning can underestimate the presence and extent of pancreatic necrosis.
  - o Dilation of the CBD alone is neither sensitive nor specific for the diagnosis of CBD stones.

2. After 48 hours
  - Laboratory
    - o Monitor CBC, renal function, electrolytes including serum calcium, $O_2$ saturation.
    - o CRP >150 mg/dL suggests severe pancreatitis (sensitivity of 80%, specificity of 76%, PPV of 67%, and negative PV of 86%) and is strongly associated with the existence of pancreatic necrosis.[2-4]

3. After 72 hours
  - Laboratory
    - o Monitor CBC, renal function, electrolytes including serum calcium, $O_2$ saturation.

- Imaging
  - Abdominal CT scan with rapid-bolus IV contrast in patients with evidence of organ failure or those with predicted severe disease (eg, systemic inflammatory response syndrome [SIRS], Acute Physiology and Chronic Health Evaluation [APACHE] ≥8) after 72 hours.
    - Evaluate for necrosis and complications such as fluid collections.
    - Ductal disruption best seen on endoscopic retrograde cholangiopancreatography (ERCP) or less commonly magnetic resonance cholangiopancreatography (MRCP), peripancreatic vascular thromboses can be seen in different modalities.
    - Note that a CT performed within the first 72 hours of the disease process might not accurately demonstrate the degree of pancreatic necrosis.
  - Assessing etiology
    - MRCP or endoscopic ultrasonography (EUS) can accurately assess for cholelithiasis and/or choledocholithiasis.
    - MRCP and EUS are superior to CT for diagnosis of choledocholithiasis and pancreatic ductal anatomy.
    - MRCP is currently the test of choice because it is less invasive than EUS; however, if a patient is undergoing EUS, an ERCP can be performed during the same procedure if a CBD stone is detected.
    - CT scan recommended in patients with pancreatitis of unknown etiology who are older than 40 years of age to exclude an underlying pancreatic malignancy.
    - MRCP, EUS, or ERCP in patients with idiopathic pancreatitis is useful to evaluate for calculous disease of the CBD, underlying chronic pancreatitis, anatomic etiologies

(eg, pancreas divisum), or malignancy (eg, pancreatic cancer, ampullary tumor, intraductal papillary mucinous neoplasm, etc).[6]

# Assessment of Initial Disease Severity

- The majority of patients have self-limited "mild" disease with symptom improvement and full recovery within several days. Nevertheless, there is still an estimated overall mortality of 5% to 10%. During the first 2 weeks, most deaths are due to multisystem organ failure from the overwhelming inflammatory response with release of inflammatory mediators and cytokines. Late death is usually attributed to local or systemic infection.

- Stratify patients into mild or severe with clinical criteria:
  - The most accurate estimate of prognosis from AP is determined using a combination of abdominal imaging, well-established clinical scoring systems, as well as ongoing clinical assessment.[1-5]
    - "Mild" (80% to 90%) AP is associated with minimal organ dysfunction and an uneventful recovery. Usually, normal enhancement of pancreatic parenchyma on CECT.
    - "Severe" (10% to 20%) AP is associated with organ failure and/or local complications such as necrosis.
      - Consider transfer to the ICU in patients with predicted or actual severe disease.
      - Clinical predictors of a poor outcome include severe comorbid illnesses, older age, and obesity.
      - Pleural effusion on chest x-ray within the first 24 hours correlates with severity.
      - BUN elevation on admission or a rise during the first 24 hours of admission is associated with increased mortality.

**Table 7-1.**

## SYSTEMIC INFLAMMATORY
## RESPONSE SYNDROME CRITERIA

| Heart rate | >90 beats/minute |
|---|---|
| Temperature | >38°C or <36°C |
| White blood cell count | >12,000 or <4000 cells/μL or >10% bands |
| Respiratory status | Respiratory rate >20/min or $PaCO_2$ <32 mm Hg |

- ◦ Hemoconcentration with elevated Hct ≥44 on admission has been variably predictive of severe pancreatitis. The absence of hemoconcentration on admission or during initial 24 hours with rehydration is predictive of a benign clinical course.
- ◦ SIRS predisposes to multiple organ dysfunction and/or pancreatic necrosis. SIRS is defined by 2 or more of the criteria in Table 7-1 for more than 48 hours.
- ◦ APACHE II scale can be used in the first 48 hours of diagnosis and is calculated by assigning points based on age, heart rate, temperature, respiratory rate, MAP, $PaO_2$, pH, K, Na, Cr, Hct, WBC, Glasgow Coma Scale, previous health status.
- The Atlanta Symposium defined severe AP by early prognostic signs:
  - ○ Ranson's signs of 3 or more (Table 7-2)
  - ○ APACHE II score of 8 or more
  - ○ Organ failure
    - ▪ Shock-systolic pressure less than 90 mm Hg
    - ▪ $PaO_2$ of 60 mm Hg or less

**Table 7-2.**

## RANSON'S CRITERIA FOR
## SEVERITY OF ACUTE PANCREATITIS

| AT TIME OF ADMISSION OR DIAGNOSIS | WITHIN NEXT 48 HOURS | SCORE | MORTALITY |
|---|---|---|---|
| • Age >55 years<br>• White blood cell count >16,000/mm³<br>• Blood glucose >200 mg/dL<br>• LDH >2x normal (>350 IU/L)<br>• ALT >6x normal (AST >250 IU/L) | • Decrease in hematocrit >10%<br>• Serum calcium <8 mg/dL<br>• Increase in blood urea nitrogen >5 mg/dL<br>• Arterial PO₂ <60 mm Hg<br>• Base deficit >4 mEq/L<br>• Estimated fluid sequestration >6 L | <3 (severe pancreatitis unlikely) | 1% |
| | | 3 to 5 | 10% to 20% |
| | | 6 | >50% |

- Creatinine more than 2.0 mg/L after rehydration
- Gastrointestinal bleeding more than 500 cc/24 hours (to be removed from updated Atlanta Criteria)
  o Local complications*
    - Necrosis
    - Abscess
    - Pseudocyst

*Necrosis carries a greater level of importance and PV for severity of pancreatitis than corresponding late complications of abscess or pseudocyst formation.

**Table 7-3.**

## COMPUTED TOMOGRAPHY SEVERITY INDEX FOR ACUTE PANCREATITIS*

| CT FINDING GRADE | SCORE | NECROSIS SCORE | SCORE |
|---|---|---|---|
| A: Normal pancreas | 0 | None | 0 |
| B: Enlargement of the pancreas | 1 | One-third | 2 |
| C: Peripancreatic inflammatory changes | 2 | One-half | 4 |
| D: A single, ill-defined fluid collection | 3 | >One-half | 6 |
| E: Two or multiple fluid collections | 4 | | |

*CT severity index equals the combined CT finding grade score and necrosis score. The maximum score is 10. Severe disease defined by a combined score of 6 or greater.

- Stratify into mild or severe with imaging criteria (Table 7-3).
  - Distinguish between interstitial and necrotizing pancreatitis as it provides important prognostic information.
  - Interstitial pancreatitis: Defined by an intact microcirculation. On CT, this is demonstrated by uniform enhancement of the pancreas.
    - 85% of patients have interstitial disease
    - 10% of patients with interstitial disease experience organ failure, and the mortality rate is 3%
  - Necrotizing pancreatitis: Defined as diffuse or focal areas of nonviable pancreatic parenchyma due to disruption of the pancreatic microcirculation. Often associated with peripancreatic fat necrosis. On CT, this is demonstrated by large areas of the pancreas that do not enhance (>3 cm in size or >30% of the pancreas).

- 33% of patients with necrotizing pancreatitis developed infected necrosis.
- The mortality rate for necrosis is approximately 15% (30% if infected and 10% if sterile).
- Accounts for more than 50% of deaths from AP.

o MRI with gadolinium can be used for patients with contraindications to a CT scan (contrast allergy).

## INITIAL RESUSCITATION

- Fluids[2,7]
  - o "Vigorous" fluid resuscitation beginning immediately upon admission is important to reduce complications of necrosis and/or organ failure.
  - o There is no consensus as to the best rate, type, and volume of initial resuscitation as there are no prospective controlled trials to support specific recommendations in preventing complications.
  - o Crystalloid (normal saline or Lactated Ringer's) is recommended in most instances. Colloid may be considered with packed red blood cells if the hematocrit falls below 25% and albumin if the serum albumin level drops to less than 2 g/dL.
  - o Based on expert opinion and the AGA guidelines, patients with severe volume depletion should be resuscitated with 500 to 1000 mL/hr, patients with signs of extracellular fluid loss (not severe) should be initiated at a rate of 300 to 500 mL/hr, and those without volume depletion at a rate of 250 to 350 mL/hr.
  - o Adequate fluid resuscitation should achieve a urine output of more than 0.5 mL/kg/hr in the absence of renal failure.
  - o Adjustment of fluids is made every several hours based on hemodynamic and volume status.

- Correct electrolyte and metabolic abnormalities.
- Supplemental oxygen is recommended initially for all patients.
- Pain control
  - Although there is a theoretical concern of sphincter of Oddi spasm from morphine, there is no evidence to support that it should be contraindicated in patients with AP.
  - Consider patient-controlled analgesia. This approach has not been compared prospectively to on-demand analgesia.
- Nutrition
  - Nothing by mouth until the patient is pain-free, no longer requires pain medications, and develops an appetite; when oral nutrition is started, it should begin with a liquid diet and advance as tolerated. Those patients with mild disease may consider initiating oral intake with a solid, low-fat diet.
  - Initiate enteral nutrition in patients unlikely to start oral intake within 5 to 7 days.
    - Enteral nasojejunal feeding is preferred over total parenteral nutrition because it has been shown to be associated with a decreased length of stay and fewer infectious complications in patients with severe AP. It is uncertain if nasogastric (NG) feeding is a safe alternative.
    - An elemental diet (meaning a diet with amino acids, fats, sugars, vitamins, and minerals but without whole or partial protein) has been shown to reduce pancreatic stimulation by about 50% as compared to other complex formulas.
- Pharmacologic intervention
  - There are no studies to support the effectiveness of enzyme inhibitors (eg, aprotinin, gabexate mesilate) or putting the pancreas to rest (eg,

somatostatin, calcitonin, glucagon, NG suction, H2 receptor blocker) in lowering morbidity and mortality.

## MONITORING AND EVALUATING RESPONSE TO INITIAL RESUSCITATION

- Serial bedside assessments to continuously follow the patient's response to therapy and make the appropriate changes in management are critical during the initial 24 to 72 hours.
  - o Assess change in symptoms such as pain, abdominal tenderness, nausea, or vomiting.
  - o Assess intravascular volume status with orthostatics and urine output.
  - o Assess SIRS with the temperature, pulse, respirations, and leukocytosis.
- Determine if a step-up in therapy is required.
  - o If after 72 hours there is evidence of organ dysfunction (defined by partial pressure of $O_2$ <60 mm Hg, $O_2$ <90%, systolic blood pressure <90 mm Hg, creatinine >2.0 g/dL); if there is persistent pain, fever, or SIRS; or in patients with an APACHE II score of 8 or more:
    - Consider transfer to the ICU.
    - Investigate for other sources of infection (blood, urine cultures, and chest x-ray).

## DETERMINE THE ETIOLOGY OF PANCREATITIS

- Obtain a focused history: gallstones are the etiology in 45%, alcohol 35%, miscellaneous causes 10%, and idiopathic 10% to 20% (Table 7-4).

**Table 7-4.**

## CAUSES OF ACUTE PANCREATITIS

| | |
|---|---|
| Obstructive causes | Gallstones, tumors (ampullary or pancreatic tumors), parasites (ascaris or *Clonorchis*), developmental anomalies (pancreas divisum, choledochocele, annular pancreas), periampullary duodenal diverticula, hypertensive sphincter of Oddi, afferent duodenal loop obstruction |
| Toxins | Ethyl alcohol, methyl alcohol, scorpion venom (seen mostly in West Indies), organophosphorus insecticides |
| Drugs | Definite association: Azathioprine/6-mercaptopurine, valproic acid, estrogens, tetracycline, metronidazole, nitrofurantoin, pentamidine, furosemide, sulfonamides, methyldopa, cytarabine, cimetidine, ranitidine, sulindac, dideoxycytidine<br><br>Probable association: Thiazides, ethacrynic acid, phenformin, procainamide, chlorthalidone, L-asparaginase |
| Metabolic causes | Hypertriglyceridemia, hypercalcemia, end-stage renal disease |
| Trauma | Accidental: Blunt trauma to abdomen<br>Iatrogenic: Postoperative, ERCP, endoscopic sphincterotomy, sphincter of Oddi manometry |
| Infectious | Parasitic: Ascariasis, clonorchiasis<br>Viral: Mumps, rubella, hepatitis A, hepatitis B, non-A and non-B hepatitis, coxsackievirus B, echo, adenovirus, cytomegalovirus, varicella, Epstein-Barr, human immunodeficiency virus<br>Bacterial: Mycoplasma, *Campylobacter jejuni*, tuberculosis, Legionella, Leptospirosis |

*(continued)*

**Table 7-4. (continued)**

## CAUSES OF ACUTE PANCREATITIS

| | |
|---|---|
| Vascular | Ischemia: Hypoperfusion (such as post-cardiac surgery) or atherosclerotic emboli<br><br>Vasculitis: Systemic lupus erythematous, polyarteritis nodosa, malignant hypertension |
| Idiopathic | 10% to 30% of patients with pancreatitis. Up to 60% of these patients have occult gallstone disease (biliary microlithiasis or gallbladder sludge). Other less common causes include sphincter of Oddi dysfunction, mutations in the cystic fibrosis transmembrane regulator |
| Miscellaneous | Penetrating peptic ulcer, Crohn's disease of the duodenum, pregnancy associated, pediatric association (Reye's syndrome, cystic fibrosis) |

- o Symptoms of biliary colic characterized by rapid onset steady right upper quadrant pain; last 30 minutes to several hours; and are sometimes associated with nausea, vomiting, and occasional radiation to the shoulder, back, or flank.
- o Prior imaging documenting gallstones.
- o History of alcohol use.
- o Medication history (both prescription and non-prescription).
- o Laboratory studies: Hypertriglyceridemia, hypercalcemia.
  - ▪ A 3-fold elevation in ALT has a 95% PPV for biliary pancreatitis.
- o Family history of pancreatitis.
- o History of autoimmune diseases.
- o History of trauma including abdominal and iatrogenic such as post-ERCP.

# THERAPEUTIC PLANS FOR THE PROBLEM

## MANAGEMENT OF THE MORE COMMON ETIOLOGIES

- Gallstone pancreatitis[1-5]
    - Noninvasive imaging (see imaging section discussed previously).
    - ERCP indicated for choledocholithiasis, as determined by MRCP or EUS, or if there is a high suspicion of an impacted stone based on labs:
        - Urgent (within 24 hours): For suspected cholangitis.
        - Early (within 72 hours): For those with a high suspicion of a retained CBD stone (based on imaging by MRCP or EUS or jaundice).
    - Cholecystectomy
        - Obtain a surgical consult for timing of cholecystectomy.
        - Cholecystectomy should be performed in the same hospital admission if possible or, otherwise, no later than 2 to 4 weeks after discharge. This is based on a high incidence of early recurrent episodes of pancreatitis (up to 30%).
    - Nonsurgical candidates
        - Consider ERCP with sphincterotomy.
- Alcohol use, prescription and nonprescription drugs
    - Avoidance.
    - Referral to counseling services.
- Hypertriglyceridemia
    - Hypertriglyceridemia-induced AP is usually seen with triglyceride levels higher than 1000 mg/dL.
    - There are case series on the acute treatment of hypertriglyceridemia with combined heparin and insulin, which induce lipoprotein lipase;

apheresis has also been used but there are no prospective trials.

- o Lipid- and triglyceride-lowering medications as an outpatient.
- Hypercalcemia
  - o Medical therapy to normalize serum calcium.
  - o Determine the etiology (ie, hyperparathyroidism, neoplasm, familial hypocalciuric hypercalcemia).
  - o Note that Lactated Ringer's is contraindicated as it has 3 mEq/L of calcium.

## MANAGEMENT OF LOCAL COMPLICATIONS

- Acute fluid collections: Collections of fluid in and adjacent to the pancreas are common in patients with severe pancreatitis.
  - o Acute fluid collections are defined as localized pancreatic fluid, without solid components, located near the pancreas. They occur with interstitial or necrotizing pancreatitis and always lack a wall of granulation tissue.
    - Most are absorbed spontaneously within the first several weeks after the onset of AP.
    - Rarely require intervention unless they become infected, which is infrequent.
  - o A pancreatic pseudocyst is a mature fluid collection present for a minimum of 4 weeks. In symptomatic patients, if the pseudocyst is mature and encapsulated, treatment can involve endoscopic, surgical, and percutaneous drainage.
- Infected pancreatic necrosis: This is a strong determinant of the severity of illness and accounts for a large percentage of the deaths from AP. It should be suspected in patients with persistent symptoms of abdominal pain, persistent fever or SIRS, or organ dysfunction after 72 hours.

o Prophylactic antibiotics: Guidelines are equivocal on the use of prophylactic antibiotics as recent double-blind, placebo-controlled trials and a meta-analysis failed to demonstrate any benefit for prevention of infection in necrotizing pancreatitis. If used, the AGA guideline suggests restricting to patients with substantial necrosis (>30% of the pancreas) and limiting duration to less than 14 days.[2]

o Diagnosis: CT-guided fine needle aspiration of the necrosis obtained for gram stain and culture. This technique is safe and accurate for diagnosis of infected necrosis. Antibiotics may be started prior to diagnosis of infected necrosis. The choice should take into consideration those that penetrate into the pancreas, such as imipenem-cilastatin, meropenem, or a combination of a quinolone and metronidazole. Once culture results are available, the antibiotics can be tailored, or if negative for infection, they can be discontinued.

o Treatment: There is consensus that the best outcomes are achieved when surgery is delayed until approximately 4 weeks after the onset of pancreatitis to allow for liquefaction. Traditional management of infected pancreatic necrosis typically involves surgical débridement with necrosectomy and closed irrigation via indwelling catheters, necrosectomy with closed drainage without irrigation, or necrosectomy and open packing.

A more conservative "step-up" approach is gaining favor in which percutaneous drainage is the initial treatment. If this initial approach fails, it is followed by a less invasive video-assisted retroperitoneal débridement.[8]

- Other complications of AP that are beyond the scope of the current discussion include pancreatic ductal disruption, arterial pseudoaneurysm formation, peripancreatic vascular thrombosis (splenic vein, portal vein, and superior mesenteric vein), and exocrine or endocrine insufficiency.

# SUMMARY ALGORITHM FOR THE MANAGEMENT OF ACUTE PANCREATITIS

## Key Points

- The diagnosis of AP is made if 2 of the following criteria are met: characteristic abdominal pain, serum amylase or lipase more than 3 times normal, or characteristic findings on abdominal imaging (CT or MRI).
- CT scanning is not necessary as an initial test if the diagnosis of AP is clear; an ultrasound, however, is useful to identify cholelithiasis and CBD dilation.
- Stratification of patients into "mild" or "severe" pancreatitis has important implications for prognosis. This can be done via scoring systems (APACHE, Ranson's, Atlanta), simple clinical features (hemoconcentration, presence of SIRS), or CT-based criteria.
- The mainstay of therapy is aggressive fluid resuscitation. Medical teams often fail to hydrate patients appropriately for fear of inducing volume overload, but current guidelines suggest at least 250 to 350 mL/hr of crystalloid infusion even if volume depletion is not evident. If volume depletion is severe, infusion rates of 500 to 1000 mL/hr are recommended.
- Patients with AP should remain NPO (nothing by mouth) until they are pain free and need no analgesics. If a patient remains NPO for more than 5 to 7 days, consider nasojejunal feeding.

*(continued)*

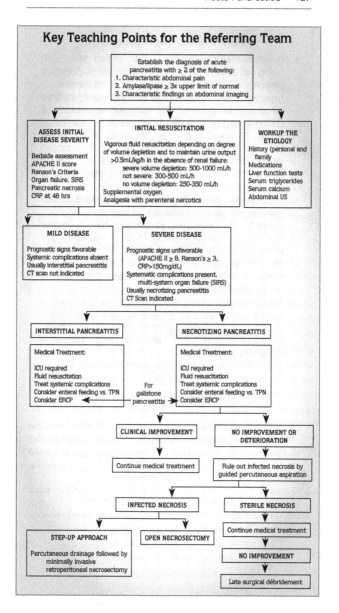

**Key Teaching Points for the Referring Team**

Establish the diagnosis of acute pancreatitis with ≥ 2 of the following:
1. Characteristic abdominal pain
2. Amylase/lipase ≥ 3x upper limit of normal
3. Characteristic findings on abdominal imaging

**ASSESS INITIAL DISEASE SEVERITY**

Bedside assessment
APACHE II score
Ranson's Criteria
Organ failure, SIRS
Pancreatic necrosis
CRP at 48 hrs

**INITIAL RESUSCITATION**

Vigorous fluid resuscitation depending on degree of volume depletion and to maintain urine output >0.5mL/kg/h in the absence of renal failure:
severe volume depletion: 500-1000 mL/h
not severe: 300-500 mL/h
no volume depletion: 250-350 mL/h
Supplemental oxygen
Analgesia with parenteral narcotics

**WORKUP THE ETIOLOGY**

History (personal and family)
Medications
Liver function tests
Serum triglycerides
Serum calcium
Abdominal US

**MILD DISEASE**

Prognostic signs favorable
Systemic complications absent
Usually interstitial pancreatitis
CT scan not indicated

**SEVERE DISEASE**

Prognostic signs unfavorable
(APACHE II ≥ 8, Ranson's ≥ 3, CRP>150mg/dL)
Systematic complications present, multi-system organ failure (SIRS)
Usually necrotizing pancreatitis
CT Scan indicated

**INTERSTITIAL PANCREATITIS**

Medical Treatment:
ICU required
Fluid resuscitation
Treat systemic complications
Consider enteral feeding vs. TPN
Consider ERCP

For gallstone pancreatitis

**NECROTIZING PANCREATITIS**

Medical Treatment:
ICU required
Fluid resuscitation
Treat systemic complications
Consider enteral feeding vs. TPN
Consider ERCP

**CLINICAL IMPROVEMENT**

Continue medical treatment

**NO IMPROVEMENT OR DETERIORATION**

Rule out infected necrosis by guided percutaneous aspiration

**INFECTED NECROSIS**

**STERILE NECROSIS**

Continue medical treatment

**STEP-UP APPROACH**

Percutaneous drainage followed by minimally invasive retroperitoneal necrosectomy

**OPEN NECROSECTOMY**

**NO IMPROVEMENT**

Late surgical débridement

## *Key Points (continued)*

- Evaluation of the etiology of AP should start with ruling out alcoholic and gallstone pancreatitis (together responsible for 80% of AP). Next, hypertriglyceridemia, hypercalcemia, autoimmune AP, and drug-induced AP should be explored. For gallstone pancreatitis, if choledocholithiasis is identified, ERCP is warranted within 72 hours and within 24 hours in suspected cholangitis to remove impacted stones or to establish biliary drainage. The value of ERCP for severe pancreatitis in the absence of biliary obstruction is unknown.
- Patients who fail to improve within 72 hours should have a contrast CT to evaluate for pancreatic necrosis. Patients with necrotizing pancreatitis have a greater risk of multi-organ system failure and a higher mortality. Needle aspiration of the pancreas to look for infected necrosis should be considered if the patient fails to improve or worsens after 3 to 7 days of conservative therapy.
- The possible complications of acute pancreatitis include, but are not limited to, fluid collections, ductal disruption, peripancreatic vascular thrombosis, pseudoaneurysm, and exocrine and endocrine dysfunction.

# REFERENCES

1. American Gastroenterological Association (AGA) Institute on "Management of Acute Pancreatitis" Clinical Practice and Economics Committee; AGA Institute Governing Board. AGA Institute medical position statement on acute pancreatitis. *Gastroenterology.* 2007;132:2019-2021.
2. Forsmark CE, Baillie J. AGA Institute technical review on acute pancreatitis. *Gastroenterology.* 2007;132:2022-2044.
3. Banks PA, Freeman ML. Practice guidelines in acute pancreatitis. *Am J Gastroenterol.* 2006;101:2379-2400.

4.  Working Party of the British Society of Gastroenterology; Association of Surgeons of Great Britain and Ireland; Pancreatic Society of Great Britain and Ireland; Association of Upper GI Surgeons of Great Britain and Ireland. UK guidelines for the management of acute pancreatitis. *Gut.* 2005;54(suppl 3):iii1-iii9.

5.  Otsuki M, Hirota M, Arata S, et al. Consensus of primary care in acute pancreatitis in Japan. *World J Gastroenterol.* 2006;12:3314-3323.

6.  Adler DG, Baron TH, Davila RE, et al. ASGE guideline: the role of ERCP in diseases of the biliary tract and the pancreas. *Gastrointest Endosc.* 2005;62:1-8.

7.  Gardner TB, Vege SS, Pearson RK, et al. Fluid resuscitation in acute pancreatitis. *Clin Gastroenterol Hepatol.* 2008;6:1070-1076.

8.  van Santvoort HC, Besselink MG, Bakker OJ, et al. A step-up approach or open necrosectomy for necrotizing pancreatitis. *N Engl J Med.* 2010;362:1491-1502.

# 8

# Acute Cholangitis and Biliary Emergencies

Stephen D. Humm, MD
Christopher S. Huang, MD

You receive the following call from the emergency department:

*A 67-year-old obese mother of 3 with a history of diabetes and hypertension presented to the emergency room tonight with abdominal pain, nausea, and vomiting. Her pain began suddenly this afternoon after eating a hamburger. The pain is in the right upper quadrant, radiating to her back and right shoulder. She has had similar, milder attacks in the past. On physical examination, she is tender to palpation on the right upper quadrant, but she does not appear to have an acute abdomen.*

The most common biliary emergencies that gastroenterologists encounter are those related to gallstone disease, namely choledocholithiasis, acute cholangitis, and gallstone pancreatitis. The classic scenario is a patient as described in the case vignette presenting with acute, severe epigastric or right upper quadrant pain, radiating to the back or right shoulder/scapula and often associated with nausea and vomiting.

Lowe RC, Farraye FA.
*GI Emergencies: A Quick Reference Guide* (pp 131-146).
© 2012 Taylor & Francis Group

The first step after obtaining the history and performing the physical examination is to generate a differential diagnosis.

## DIFFERENTIAL DIAGNOSIS

- Biliary colic: Pain due to transient obstruction of the cystic duct; despite the name "colic," this pain is NOT colicky (waxing/waning in waves), but rather a steady and persistent pain that plateaus for a variable amount of time before abating.
- Acute cholecystitis: Inflammation of the gallbladder due to persistent obstruction of the cystic duct, frequently complicated by infection.
- Choledocholithiasis: Common bile duct (CBD) stones.
- Pancreatitis.
- Acute hepatitis.
- Peptic ulcer.
- Myocardial ischemia: Particularly inferior wall or right ventricular.
- Aortic dissection or expansion/rupture of an abdominal aortic aneurysm.
- Pneumonia: Typically right lower or middle lobe.

*As you hear the story and generate a differential, you realize that you need additional information to confirm a diagnosis and effectively triage this patient. In particular, does this patient need an emergency endoscopic retrograde cholangiopancreatography (ERCP)?*

## INITIAL TESTING

Initial diagnostic testing should include a complete blood count (CBC), liver chemistries, amylase, lipase, cardiac enzymes, electrocardiogram, and chest x-ray. Blood cultures should be obtained when there are signs of infection, and coagulation studies should be checked.

An abdominal ultrasound (US) is the diagnostic test of choice for initial evaluation of patients with suspected gallstone disease. A computed tomography (CT) scan of the abdomen and pelvis may be best if the diagnosis is unclear, or if a severe intra-abdominal catastrophe (eg, perforation) is suspected.

# INDICATIONS FOR URGENT ENDOSCOPIC RETROGRADE CHOLANGIOPANCREATOGRAPHY IN PATIENTS WITH GALLSTONE DISEASE

Once it has been determined that the patient indeed has a gallstone-related problem, you should try to estimate the likelihood that there is an obstructing stone in the bile duct (see below) and decide whether early ERCP is indicated.[1] As a general rule, there is no indication for ERCP in patients with biliary colic or acute cholecystitis in the absence of concomitant CBD stones, cholangitis, or Mirizzi's syndrome. Patients with CBD stones should undergo ERCP, the timing of which can be guided by the patient's condition and whether cholangitis is present. Most patients with gallstone pancreatitis do not need (or benefit from) early ERCP. Although controversial, some evidence suggests that patients with severe gallstone pancreatitis may benefit from early biliary intervention. Of the gallstone-related problems, the only true emergency is acute cholangitis unresponsive to antibiotics and supportive measures.

*The surgical resident tells you that her initial lab results are as follows: aspartate aminotransferase (AST) 175 U/L, alanine aminotransferase (ALT) 170 U/L, total bilirubin 4 mg/dL, and alkaline phosphatase 300 U/L. Her white blood cell (WBC) is 14,000 with a "left shift." In addition, her abdominal US showed a 1.7 cm CBD with stones in her gallbladder, without signs of cholecystitis. No stones were seen in the CBD. She is febrile to 101°F and appears diaphoretic and somewhat lethargic. Her systolic blood pressure is 90 (her baseline is in the 130s), and heart rate is 100.*

It now appears that this patient has acute cholangitis and features of sepsis. Based on her clinical appearance, she will require close monitoring (ICU admission), immediate initiation of IV fluids and broad-spectrum antibiotics, and potentially an urgent ERCP.

# ACUTE CHOLANGITIS

Acute cholangitis is a bacterial infection of the biliary tree that results from impaired biliary drainage, leading to systemic signs of infection.

- Pathophysiology: Normally, bile is sterile and bacteriostatic. When obstruction develops, normal biliary defense mechanisms are overwhelmed, allowing bacteria from the duodenum or the portal circulation to seed the biliary tract and lead to infection. CBD stones are the leading cause of cholangitis.
- Most common organisms: Gram-negatives (*E. coli, Klebsiella,* or *Enterobacter*), gram-positives (especially *Enterococcus*), and anaerobes (*Clostridium*).

## DIAGNOSIS

- Clinical presentation
  - Charcot's triad: Classic presentation for cholangitis (present in approximately 50% to 75% of cases) with fever, abdominal pain, and jaundice.
  - Reynold's pentad: Charcot's Triad + hypotension and altered mental status indicates "pus under pressure."
- Laboratory abnormalities
  - Leukocytosis with left-shift.

- o Conjugated hyperbilirubinemia, elevated alkaline phosphatase (typical of extrahepatic bile duct obstruction).
  - o ALT and AST elevation is variable. Although not typical, transient extreme transaminase elevation (into the 1000s range) can be seen in "postobstructive hepatitis."
  - o Blood cultures are positive in approximately 50% of patients.
- Imaging: Abdominal US will typically demonstrate dilation of the intrahepatic and/or extrahepatic bile ducts, indicating mechanical obstruction. The normal CBD size is 3 to 6 mm in diameter but increases with age (approximately 1 mm for each decade of life). The CBD can also be enlarged in someone who is status post-CCY (up to 1 cm). US is very sensitive for detecting bile duct dilation and is specific, but not sensitive, for CBD stones. Therefore, in the patient presenting with clinical and biochemical signs of severe cholangitis, the absence of bile duct stones on US does not rule out the diagnosis. In stable patients with clinically mild cholangitis, CT or magnetic resonance cholangiopancreatography (MRCP) can be helpful if the US findings are equivocal. However, in patients with severe cholangitis, further imaging must not delay biliary drainage.

## MANAGEMENT

- The 3 key aspects of cholangitis management are resuscitation, adequate antibiotic therapy, and biliary decompression.[2]
- Resuscitation: The first step in any patient with suspected cholangitis is aggressive hydration and resuscitation. In the majority of cases, the patient will respond and stabilize. Only if the patient does not respond appropriately is urgent/emergent decompression necessary. Ensure that the patient has adequate venous access as you would in any acutely ill patient.

- Antibiotic coverage—Initial coverage should be broad and should provide therapy for all of the organisms listed previously. Although there are no firm guidelines on the antibiotic therapy for cholangitis, a variety of options are available.
  - Two common options would be a third-generation cephalosporin or a fluoroquinolone with or without metronidazole. Alternatively, monotherapy with a carbapenem is an option.
  - Blood cultures should be sent on admission, and cultures of aspirated bile can also be obtained during ERCP. Antibiotics should then be tailored based on culture data. Please note that cultures from blood and bile may not always yield the same organism, which can complicate the decision as to which antibiotic treatment is optimal.
  - No firm guidelines exist regarding the optimal duration of antibiotic treatment. A short course (2 to 3 days) may be sufficient for patients with mild cholangitis, but a 5- to 7-day course is typically used for moderate-to-severe cholangitis.
- Biliary decompression: Most patients will respond to resuscitation and antimicrobial therapy. However, definitive therapy requires restoration of bile flow. This can be accomplished endoscopically, percutaneously, or surgically. ERCP with endoscopic sphincterotomy (ES) and stone clearance is the preferred method, although ERCP with temporary stent placement or percutaneous approaches can be used in very unstable patients. Surgery now has no role in the management of acute cholangitis.
  - ERCP/ES: This is the preferred method for biliary decompression. The urgency of the procedure depends largely on the patient's clinical stability. If the patient responds well to hydration and broad-spectrum antibiotics, the procedure can be done more electively (usually in 24 to 48 hours). However, if the patient remains acutely ill, a more urgent procedure may be required.

- Indications for urgent ERCP: Hypotension, persistent fevers, and altered mental status despite resuscitation and antibiotics.
- Remember that if a temporary stent is placed, the patient will need a follow-up procedure in 4 to 6 weeks to remove the stent and complete stone clearance.
- Key point: Match your intervention to the acuity of the case. Resuscitation and antibiotics come first. However, if the patient doesn't stabilize, then he or she may have "pus under pressure" and may need a procedure overnight or first thing in the morning.
  ○ Percutaneous drainage: Although ERCP is preferred over percutaneous biliary drainage, the latter approach may be required for patients who fail initial ERCP or for those with abnormal postsurgical anatomy (eg, Roux-en-Y) when an endoscopist with expertise in the management of postsurgical patients is not available or if the patient is too unstable to endure a potentially prolonged and unsuccessful ERCP.

*Let's say instead that when the surgical resident calls you, the patient is in fact afebrile and well-appearing with a normal WBC. The liver function tests and US findings are abnormal as previously described.*

This patient still has signs of biliary obstruction. However, the key difference is that she is not manifesting any signs of infection. The most likely cause for her presentation is an obstructing stone in her CBD—choledocholithiasis.

## CHOLEDOCHOLITHIASIS

- Choledocholithiasis is most commonly suspected in patients with symptomatic cholelithiasis and acute gallstone pancreatitis. A combination of readily

**Table 8-1.**

### PREDICTORS OF CHOLEDOCHOLITHIASIS

| Very strong | CBD stone seen on US<br>Clinical ascending cholangitis<br>Bilirubin >4 mg/dL |
| --- | --- |
| Strong | Dilated CBD on US >6 mm (with gallbladder in situ)<br>Bilirubin level 1.8 to 4 mg/dL |
| Moderate | Abnormal liver biochemical test (besides bilirubin)<br>Age >55 years<br>Clinical gallstone pancreatitis |

available clinical, biochemical, and radiographic data can be used to categorize patients as having a low (<10%), intermediate (10% to 50%), or high (>50%) probability of having CBD stones. Patients have a high likelihood of CBD stones if any very strong predictor or both strong predictors are present (Table 8-1). Conversely, they have a low likelihood if no predictors are present, and all others can be categorized as intermediate risk. Management decisions can then be guided by the patient's risk category (Figure 8-1).[3]

## DIAGNOSIS

- Clinical presentation
  - Similar to that of patients with biliary colic/cholecystitis, with the possible addition of scleral icterus, bilirubinuria, or acholic stools.
- Laboratory abnormalities
  - Conjugated hyperbilirubinemia, elevated alkaline phosphatase—these cholestatic liver biochemical tests generally increase progressively with the duration and severity of obstruction. However, fewer than one-third of patients will have a bilirubin greater than 4 mg/dL.

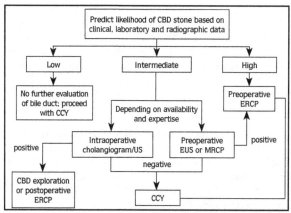

**Figure 8-1.** Management algorithm for patients with possible CBD stone.

- ○ ALT, AST elevation is variable. Although not typical, transient extreme transaminase elevation (into the 1000s range) can be seen in acute postobstructive hepatitis due to CBD stones.
- ○ Keep in mind that, typically, alkaline phosphatase and bilirubin are elevated in cases of biliary obstruction. However, the transaminases may be the first to rise in the acute setting, and the other values may lag behind.
- ○ Completely normal panel of liver biochemistries has a very high negative predictive value (~97%).
- Imaging: As mentioned above, transabdominal US has a poor sensitivity for detecting CBD stones (25% to 60%), and the distal CBD is often difficult to visualize due to air in overlying loops of bowel. However, US reliably detects ductal dilatation, and a dilated CBD of >6 mm (with gallbladder in situ) is a strong predictor of CBD stones. CT scan (especially helical CT) is more sensitive than US, but its use as a first-line test for CBD stones has been limited

by expense and radiation exposure. Depending on local expertise and available technology, endoscopic ultrasound (EUS) and MRCP are extremely sensitive (85% to 95%) and specific (95% to 97%) for detecting CBD stones (although sensitivity of MRCP for stones <6 mm in size is lower, ranging from 33% to 70%).

## MANAGEMENT

Figure 8-1 depicts a suggested management algorithm for patients with symptomatic cholelithiasis and possible CBD stone. The first step is to risk-stratify the patient (low, intermediate, or high risk of CBD stone) based on clinical, laboratory, and radiographic findings (see Table 8-1).

- Low-risk patient
  - No further evaluation prior to cholecystectomy (CCY) is recommended.
- Intermediate-risk patient
  - Further evaluation is recommended to determine the need for duct clearance prior to CCY. Because of the risks of ERCP, less invasive testing is preferable. Depending on local expertise, good options include preoperative EUS or MRCP; alternatively, intraoperative cholangiogram (IOC) or laparoscopic US can be considered.
  - Patients with positive preoperative EUS or MRCP should undergo preoperative ERCP.
  - Patients with a positive IOC or laparoscopic US should undergo CBD exploration (depending on expertise of the surgeon) or postoperative ERCP.
- High-risk patient
  - Preoperative ERCP is typically recommended for these patients. The timing of ERCP depends on the clinical scenario: in the absence of severe cholangitis, ERCP can be performed electively when experienced nursing staff and technicians are available.

- In patients with clinical signs of cholangitis, antibiotics should be administered. Otherwise, patients with CBD stones do not routinely need antibiotics. However, case-by-case exceptions to this rule can be made if there is undue delay before stone extraction can be performed, and the patient is frail or has multiple comorbidities.

*Wisely, when the surgical resident initially called you, you requested that amylase and lipase be checked. These values are now back, and both are in the 1000s.*

# GALLSTONE PANCREATITIS

- Gallstone pancreatitis is thought to be triggered by impaction of a CBD stone at the ampulla of Vater, leading to pancreatic duct obstruction and the subsequent cascade of local and systemic inflammatory sequelae. Usually, gallstone pancreatitis is caused by small stones that spontaneously pass into the intestine in most cases.

## DIAGNOSIS

- Clinical presentation
  - Severe, constant epigastric or central abdominal pain, radiating "straight through" to the back, frequently accompanied by nausea/vomiting.
  - Pain may be alleviated by bending forward.
- Laboratory abnormalities
  - Amylase and lipase elevation, usually at least 3 times the upper limit of normal.
  - Transaminase elevation of at least 3 times the upper limit of normal is indicative of a biliary etiology of pancreatitis.
  - Cholestatic biochemical tests may be abnormal due to CBD obstruction from a stone or compression of the CBD secondary to pancreatic/duodenal edema.

- Imaging: In patients with a clinical presentation consistent with acute pancreatitis, combined with corroborating laboratory abnormalities, immediate imaging is not required to confirm the diagnosis. A CT scan, if performed, may demonstrate a spectrum of abnormalities, including edema of the pancreas, peripancreatic stranding, and peripancreatic fluid collections. Imaging of the bile duct to assess for CBD stones is discussed above. Both MRCP and EUS have been demonstrated to be an accurate modality for imaging the CBD in the setting of acute gallstone pancreatitis and can be used as first-line tests when therapeutic ERCP is not clearly indicated.

## MANAGEMENT

- Supportive care: Initial care is similar to treatment of any other form of acute pancreatitis, including bowel rest, pain control, and aggressive fluid resuscitation (see Chapter 7).
- Role of early ERCP: The role of early ERCP/ES in acute gallstone pancreatitis is controversial and has been an area of much interest and debate. Three randomized controlled trials in the late 1980s and mid 1990s found that ERCP performed within 24 to 72 hours of presentation significantly reduced mortality and complications from gallstone pancreatitis among patients predicted to have severe pancreatitis. However, these studies included patients with evidence of biliary obstruction and cholangitis, which are independent indications for ERCP. A Cochrane review in 2004 controlled for these confounders and still demonstrated a reduction in complications (but not mortality) in patients with predicted severe disease.[4] However, this benefit has not been confirmed in subsequent studies (randomized controlled trials and meta-analyses) involving patients without cholangitis.[5,6] Therefore, in the absence of cholangitis or

persistent CBD obstruction from a retained stone, there does not seem to be a role for early ERCP in the management of acute gallstone pancreatitis.

- CCY: Individuals who are surgically fit who have had an episode of gallstone pancreatitis should undergo CCY to prevent recurrent episodes. The optimal timing of CCY is a matter of debate and is beyond the scope of this chapter. However, CCY can be safely performed during the same hospitalization in patients with mild pancreatitis. If there is anticipated delay before CCY (particularly >2 weeks), or if the patient is not a surgical candidate, then prophylactic ERCP/ES can be offered to prevent future bouts of gallstone pancreatitis (but this will not prevent other gallstone-related problems).

*The patient eventually recovers from her acute issues and undergoes an attempted laparoscopic CCY, which is converted to an open procedure due to marked inflammation. Jackson-Pratt (JP) drains placed during her surgery have had persistent bilious drainage, and the surgery team calls you again.*

## BILE LEAKS

In the age of laparoscopic CCY, postoperative bile leaks are not uncommon (up to 1% of cases). These leaks most commonly arise from the cystic duct stump that was clipped during the operation. Alternatively, there can be a leak from the accessory duct of Luschka, which arises from the right intrahepatic duct system and drains directly into the gallbladder. Patients with a bile leak often present with pain and perhaps fever and leukocytosis shortly after a CCY. A leak can be confirmed with a hepatobiliary iminodiacetic acid scan if the diagnosis is unclear. When the diagnosis of an intraperitoneal bile leak is confirmed, external drainage via JP drains is required to prevent bile peritonitis. ERCP/ES or a stent is then indicated to ablate the pressure gradient between the biliary system and duodenum. This allows bile to preferentially flow down the "path of least resistance" into the duodenum, promoting healing of the leak. Efficacy of this procedure is excellent and can avoid the need for repeat surgery in the vast majority of cases. Most minor leaks will heal following ES alone, but stenting may be required to treat major leaks. In rare cases of persistent, major cystic duct stump leak, multiple stents placed across the cystic duct insertion site may be required.

*Another thing the surgeons may call you about...*

Traumatic bile leaks: In cases of severe penetrating or blunt-force trauma, liver injuries can occur resulting in disruption of intra- or even extra-hepatic bile ducts and subsequent free bile leak or contained bilomas. There are a few small uncontrolled studies that have shown that ERCP with ES and stent placement can be helpful in healing these injuries. As in post-CCY bile leaks, the rationale is to provide a "path of least resistance" away from the injury.

---

### Key Things to Do in Patients With a Suspected Biliary Emergency

- Generate a differential diagnosis, obtain CBC, liver biochemical panel, amylase, lipase, and abdominal US.
- Determine the likelihood of bile duct obstruction (and hence need for ERCP) using a combination of clinical, laboratory, and radiographic data.
- In patients with severe cholangitis, start broad-spectrum antibiotics and prepare for the possible need for urgent ERCP.
- Evaluate the bile duct in patients with acute gallstone pancreatitis (preferably with MRCP or EUS) to identify patients who may benefit from ERCP.

# SUMMARY

The most common biliary emergencies are caused by complications of gallstone disease, with acute cholangitis unresponsive to supportive measures being the main indication for urgent/emergent ERCP. There may be a benefit of early ERCP in patients with severe gallstone pancreatitis, although this remains an area of controversy.

---

### Key Points for the Consulting Team

- Patients demonstrating Reynold's pentad have "pus under pressure" and must be treated aggressively. Most patients will respond to fluids and antibiotics, but those who do not will require urgent ERCP.
- ERCP should be reserved for therapeutic indications only. In nonemergent situations, less invasive bile duct investigations such as MRCP or EUS can be obtained first. However, in unstable patients with cholangitis, do not waste time with further imaging.
- Most patients with acute gallstone pancreatitis do not benefit from ERCP. Only those with persistent bile duct obstruction or cholangitis have a definite indication for ERCP.

---

# REFERENCES

1. Adler DG, Baron TH, Davila RE, et al. ASGE guideline: the role of ERCP in diseases of the biliary tract and the pancreas. *Gastrointest Endosc*. 2005;62:1-7.
2. Lee JG. Diagnosis and management of acute cholangitis. *Nat Rev Gastroenterol Hepatol*. 2009;6:533-541.
3. Maple JT, Ben-Menachem T, Anderson MA, et al. The role of endoscopy in the evaluation of suspected choledocholithiasis. *Gastrointest Endosc*. 2010;71:1-9.
4. Ayub K, Slavin J, Imada R. Endoscopic retrograde cholangiopancreatography in gallstone-associated acute pancreatitis. *Cochrane Database Syst Rev*. 2004;4:CD003630.

5. Moretti A, Papi C, Aratari A, et al. Is early endoscopic retrograde cholangiopancreatography useful in the management of acute biliary pancreatitis? A meta-analysis of randomized controlled trials. *Dig Liver Dis.* 2008;40:379-385.

6. Petrov MS, van Santvoort HC, Besselink MG, et al. Early endoscopic retrograde cholangiopancreatography versus conservative management in acute biliary pancreatitis without cholangitis: a meta-analysis of randomized trials. *Ann Surg.* 2008;247:250-257.

# 9

# Evaluation and Management of Acute Liver Failure

*Rajeev Prabakaran, MD*
*Robert C. Lowe, MD*

You receive the following call from the emergency department:

*A 28-year-old man with no past medical history presents with 2 weeks of nausea, fatigue, yellowing of his skin and eyes, and dark urine. He was finally convinced by his family to come for evaluation due to worsening anorexia and increased forgetfulness.*

*Initial labs revealed: Normal complete blood count including white blood count and platelets, normal chemistries; the liver enzyme panel is remarkable for aspartate aminotransferase 1240, alanine aminotransferase 1912, alkaline phosphatase (AP) 128, total bilirubin 5.2 (direct 4.0), albumin 3.6, and international normalized ratio (INR) 1.6.*

- Based on this clinical presentation and the corresponding laboratory values, this patient has suffered acute liver failure (ALF), defined as evidence of coagulopathy and any degree of mental alteration in

Lowe RC, Farraye FA.
*GI Emergencies: A Quick Reference Guide* (pp 147-166).
© 2012 Taylor & Francis Group

**Table 9-1.**

## MOST COMMON ETIOLOGIES OF ACUTE LIVER FAILURE IN THE UNITED STATES

| Acetaminophen | 46% |
|---|---|
| Indeterminate | 14% |
| Drugs | 11% |
| Hepatitis B | 7% |
| Autoimmune | 5% |
| Ischemia | 4% |
| Hepatitis A | 3% |
| Wilson's disease | 2% |
| Other | 7% |

Adapted from Lee WM, Squires R, Nyberg SL, Doo E, Hoofnagle JH. Acute liver failure: summary of a workshop. *Hepatology*. 2008;47(4):1401-1415.

a patient without pre-existing cirrhosis and with an illness of less than 24 weeks duration.

- The term *fulminant liver failure* traditionally includes ALF within 8 weeks after the development of jaundice in a patient without a previous history of liver disease.

- As the on-call gastroenterology consult physician, assessing the patient's clinical status, particularly if there is evidence of encephalopathy and to what degree, should be the primary task. This will help direct key evaluation and decision making, including possible Intensive care unit (ICU) admission for close neurologic monitoring and whether there is a need for urgent liver transplantation evaluation.

- Clues from the history may point to the etiology of ALF. Table 9-1 reveals the most common causes of ALF in the United States, with acetaminophen, drug

**Table 9-2.**

## OTHER CAUSES OF ACUTE LIVER FAILURE

| | |
|---|---|
| Epstein-Barr virus (EBV) | Cytomegalovirus (CMV) |
| Herpes simplex virus (HSV) | Varicella zoster virus (VZV) |
| Adenovirus | Tuberculosis |
| Malignancy | Budd-Chiari syndrome |
| Congestive heart failure | Vaso-occlusive disease |
| Sepsis | Acute fatty liver of pregnancy/HELLP syndrome (hemolysis, elevated liver enzymes, low platelet count) |
| Heat stroke | Giant cell hepatitis |

injury (other than acetaminophen), and viral hepatitis the most common identifiable causes. Table 9-2 lists some of the less common etiologies for ALF.

*You proceed to the hospital. What questions should be asked of the patient to complete the history?*

- Confirm the patient's history and timeline of symptoms.
- Unearth pertinent history that may not have been addressed by the initial evaluating team, particularly a thorough prescription, over-the-counter, and herbal drug history.
- Tables 9-3 and 9-4 list some common drugs and herbal products/supplements that have been associated with liver injury leading to ALF.[1]
- Remember that in most cases, drug-induced liver failure is a diagnosis of exclusion, and other etiologies should be ruled out first.
- Confirm any risk factors for the acquisition of viral hepatitis, particularly hepatitis A and B, as hepatitis C rarely causes ALF.

**Table 9-3.**

## DRUGS ASSOCIATED WITH
## IDIOSYNCRATIC LIVER INJURY

| |
|---|
| *ANTICONVULSANTS/ANTIDEPRESSANTS* |
| Valproic acid, phenytoin, nefazodone, imipramine |
| *ANTIBIOTICS/ANTIFUNGALS/ANTIRETROVIRALS* |
| Isoniazid, bactrim, ofloxacin, augmentin, dapsone, ketoconazole, didanosine, efavirenz |
| *CARDIOVASCULAR DRUGS* |
| Labetalol, amiodarone, lisinopril, statins, nicotinic acid, methyldopa |
| *ANTIDIABETICS* |
| Troglitazone, metformin |
| *CHEMOTHERAPEUTICS* |
| Etoposide, gemtuzumab, flutamide |
| *ANESTHETICS* |
| Isoflurane, halothane |
| *RECREATIONAL DRUGS* |
| Mushrooms, amphetamines, Ecstasy, cocaine |
| *MISCELLANEOUS DRUGS* |
| Propylthiouracil, disulfiram, tolcapone, allopurinol |

- Inquire as to a personal or family history of liver or autoimmune disorders, which may predispose a patient to autoimmune hepatitis, especially in a young woman.
- A history of neuropsychiatric symptoms or movement disorders may point to Wilson's disease as an etiology. A prior history of deep vein thrombosis or other abnormal vascular thrombosis may be a clue to Budd-Chiari syndrome, as would the use of estrogen

**Table 9-4.**

## HERBAL PRODUCTS AND DIETARY SUPPLEMENTS ASSOCIATED WITH HEPATOTOXICITY

- Ma huang
- Green tea extract
- Kava kava
- Skullcap
- Pennyroyal
- Heliotrope
- Valerian
- Greater celandine
- He Shou Wu
- Chaparral
- Comfrey
- Germander
- Jin Bu Huan
- Rattleweed
- Impila
- Senecio
- Gum thistle
- Bai Fang herbs

preparations or oral contraceptives. Patients with myeloproliferative disorders are also predisposed to Budd-Chiari syndrome.

- Recreational drugs associated with ALF include cocaine, Ecstasy, and amphetamines.
- Along with a recreational drug history, inquire about mushroom ingestion, as *Amanita phalloides* can lead to ALF (very rare, but worth exploring).

*You go in to see the patient. During the encounter, he appears mildly lethargic and occasionally dozes off mid-conversation. It is late at night, but you are worried that he may be more than just sleepy. Examination also reveals a slight flapping tremor in both hands.*

- The concern now is that this patient has hepatic encephalopathy (HE) due to his liver failure, somnolence, and asterixis on examination. Stages of HE are outlined in Table 9-5.
- Other examination findings to look for include hepatomegaly or ascites from malignancy or Budd-Chiari syndrome, cervical lymphadenopathy suggestive of EBV or CMV infection, or vesicular skin lesions

**Table 9-5.**

## GRADES OF ENCEPHALOPATHY

| | |
|---|---|
| I | Changes in behavior with minimal change in level of consciousness |
| II | Gross disorientation, drowsiness, possible asterixis, inappropriate behavior |
| III | Marked confusion, incoherent speech, sleeping most of the time but arousable to vocal stimuli |
| IV | Comatose, unresponsive to pain, decorticate or decerebrate posturing |

consistent with HSV infection. The Kayser-Fleischer (K-F) rings indicative of Wilson's disease may be visible on exam, but typically require a slit-lamp examination for visualization.

- Given his encephalopathy, you should advise that the patient be admitted to a medical ICU bed to closely monitor his neurologic status, which can deteriorate rapidly. He is also provided a dose of oral lactulose.
- At this time, you should recommend the following tests to complete the initial assessment (Table 9-6): serum toxicology screen, acute viral hepatitis panel, and abdominal Doppler ultrasound, correlating with the workup of the most common etiologies.
- Other etiologies can be evaluated for if and when the above are unrevealing, or if the history or examination is suggestive of a less common cause (Table 9-7).
- Tumor infiltration of the liver is rare but can be seen with lymphoma, melanoma, breast cancer, and small cell lung cancer. Patients typically have tender hepatomegaly.

**Table 9-6.**

## INITIAL LABORATORY WORKUP
## FOR ACUTE LIVER FAILURE

- Complete blood count
- Comprehensive metabolic panel, including chemistries and renal/hepatic panels
- Prothrombin time (PT)/INR
- Arterial blood gas with lactate
- Serum ammonia level
- Toxicology screen including acetaminophen level
- Viral hepatitis serologies for hepatitis A, B, C, and E (if clinically indicated)
- Human immunodeficiency virus (HIV) testing (implications for potential liver transplantation)
- Pregnancy test for females

*Unfortunately, you are not able to obtain an accurate medication history from the patient due to his waxing/waning mental status. How should you proceed?*

- Talking with the family is essential, as they may be able to provide the missing information that can help with formulating a diagnosis and management strategy.
- They state that he is not taking any prescription medications but are unsure if he is taking any other products.
- Of interest, they do state that he was fixated on losing weight and was talking about weight loss supplements a few weeks ago.

*The abdominal Doppler ultrasound is unremarkable, with normal liver architecture and patent hepatic and portal vessels. Viral hepatitis serologies are negative for acute hepatitis A, B, and C, and hepatitis B virus (HBV) DNA is pending. Serum toxicology*

**Table 9-7.**

## WORKUP OF LESS COMMON
## CAUSES OF ACUTE LIVER FAILURE

| | |
|---|---|
| Autoimmune | Antinuclear antibody, anti-smooth muscle antibody, immunoglobulin levels; liver biopsy |
| Wilson's disease | Ceruloplasmin and serum/urine copper levels; presence of hemolytic anemia, renal failure, low AP and uric acid levels may be clues; slit-lamp evaluation for K-F rings; liver biopsy-quantitative copper level |
| Budd-Chiari syndrome | Abdominal Doppler ultrasound |
| EBV/CMV | Viral titers |
| HSV | Viral culture, liver biopsy |
| Malignant infiltration | Imaging, liver biopsy |
| Indeterminate etiology | Liver biopsy |

*screen is negative for a detectable acetaminophen level. Does this exclude acetaminophen overdose as an etiology for this liver failure?*

- An undetectable or low acetaminophen level does NOT rule out acetaminophen toxicity as the etiology for ALF, as the timing of the ingestion may not be known or remote (up to several days prior to presentation), but still can be the cause of the liver injury. Liver injury typically begins 36 hours after ingestion and peaks at around 72 hours.

- In cases with known acetaminophen ingestion, the acetaminophen toxicity nomogram may be helpful in assessing the likelihood of hepatotoxicity; it should not be used to exclude toxicity if ingestion time is unknown or when lower doses of acetaminophen are ingested, especially in patients with a history of alcohol abuse.
    - Acetaminophen toxicity is due to the production of toxic metabolites, via the cytochrome P (CYP) 450 system, that induce hepatocyte necrosis. The liver has detoxification mechanisms including sulfation, glucuronidation, and glutathione binding. High doses of acetaminophen overwhelm these protective systems.
    - Alcoholic patients have reduced sulfation and glucuronidation capabilities and reduced levels of glutathione. Moreover, alcohol induces CYP450 enzymes, leading to increased production of toxic metabolites and decreased detoxification reactions. Thus, acetaminophen hepatotoxicity can occur with lower doses of drug than in nonalcoholics.
- N-acetylcysteine (NAC), the antidote for acetaminophen poisoning, should be given in any case of ALF suspected to be due to acetaminophen. NAC works by providing antioxidant glutathione to the liver, detoxifying the acetaminophen metabolites.
- Treatment should commence as soon as possible, particularly within the first 24 hours following ingestion.
- Although no data support initiation of NAC more than 24 hours after ingestion, it is often given up to 72 hours postingestion due to its minimal side effect profile.
- If ingestion is known to have occurred less than 4 hours prior to presentation, then activated charcoal may be administered for gastrointestinal decontamination prior to NAC initiation.

*Are there any other interventions that should be done in the acute period?*

- Based on the results and the patient's possible history of dietary supplement use, you are highly suspicious for a drug/toxin-mediated liver injury.

- This fits with his pattern of hepatic panel abnormalities, and with an unremarkable serum toxicology screen, abdominal ultrasound, and acute hepatitis results, this appears to be the leading etiology. To be complete, autoimmune markers, EBV/CMV titers, ceruloplasmin, and serum and urinary copper levels are all sent and are pending.

- It is recommended that he receive NAC treatment. There is evidence that providing NAC might benefit patients with nonacetaminophen-related ALF.

  o In a recent prospective, double-blind study carried out on patients with ALF and no history of acetaminophen overdose, subjects with Grade I to II encephalopathy who received NAC had a significantly improved transplant-free survival compared to placebo.[2]

  o Notably, this benefit was not seen in Grades III to IV encephalopathy.

  o Overall, IV NAC was well-tolerated, and the study concluded that this treatment improves transplant-free survival in patients with early stage nonacetaminophen-related ALF. Those with advanced encephalopathy grades do not benefit from NAC treatment and usually require emergent liver transplantation.

  o Therefore, though it is not yet standard of care, NAC treatment for nonacetaminophen drug-induced liver failure is strongly recommended.

*Other than NAC, are there any other medical treatments for specific causes of ALF?*

- Medical treatments for other etiologies of ALF have had variable results. Table 9-8 summarizes possible options based on the etiology, if known.

**Table 9-8.**

## TREATMENT OF SPECIFIC ACUTE LIVER FAILURE ETIOLOGIES

| | |
|---|---|
| Acetaminophen | NAC; activated charcoal first if within 4 hours of presentation |
| Drug-induced | Discontinuation of offending agent; NAC |
| Viral hepatitis | Nucleoside analogues for HBV; acyclovir for HSV or VZV |
| Autoimmune hepatitis | Corticosteroids |
| Ischemic "shock" injury | Cardiovascular and hemodynamic support |
| Wilson's disease | Albumin dialysis/plasmapheresis; liver transplantation |
| Budd-Chiari syndrome | Liver transplantation (after exclusion of underlying malignancy) |
| Mushroom poisoning | Gastric lavage, activated charcoal; Penicillin G and milk thistle (silibinin)/ silymarin ± NAC; liver transplantation |
| Acute fatty liver of pregnancy/ HELLP syndrome | Expeditious delivery |

- Hepatitis B-induced ALF may benefit from new-generation nucleoside or nucleotide analogs. This is based on studies showing that early lamivudine treatment potentially prevented progression to liver transplantation.[3]
- HSV infection should be recognized and treated early with acyclovir. Although it is more likely seen in immunosuppressed and pregnant patients, it can occur in the healthy as well.

- Liver biopsy is often required for diagnosis of auto-immune-associated liver failure, as autoantibodies may be absent. Corticosteroid treatment works for some, while affected patients who fail to respond may require transplantation.

- Wilson's disease should not be treated with chelating agents (penicillamine, trientine) in the setting of ALF. Instead, albumin dialysis or plasma exchange may be initiated. Ultimately, liver transplant is typically required for survival, particularly in fulminant cases.

*When should this patient be evaluated by the liver transplant service?*

- Transplant evaluation should proceed immediately. There must not be a delay in consulting the transplant service when it comes to the diagnosis of ALF.

- This patient is critically ill with both coagulopathy and encephalopathy, and dramatic clinical deterioration can occur rapidly.

- Whether he will respond to NAC therapy is not known, and his status should be followed closely by the transplant service in case he needs to be rapidly listed for transplant.

- If the patient is not at a transplant center, planning transfer typically occurs when there is Grade I or II encephalopathy, due to the risk for swift worsening.

- Identifying possible psychosocial barriers to transplantation should be done. This includes drug or alcohol use, suicide attempts, inadequate family support, and residential status.

*Our patient has begun to receive a course of NAC, but his clinical status appears to have worsened. He is more confused, incoherent, and at times very difficult to arouse with verbal stimuli. How should our patient now be managed? What are the complications of ALF to watch for, and what are the goals of care during this ICU admission?*

**Table 9-9.**

## COMPLICATIONS OF ACUTE LIVER FAILURE

| SYSTEM INVOLVED | COMMENTS |
|---|---|
| Neurologic | Encephalopathy, cerebral edema, and elevated intracranial pressure (ICP) that can lead to herniation |
| Infectious | Bacterial and fungal, leading primarily to respiratory, urinary tract, and catheter-related infections |
| Pulmonary | Respiratory failure from metabolic disturbances or progressing encephalopathy may require airway protection and intubation with mechanical ventilation |
| Cardio-vascular | Systemic arterial vasodilatation and hypotension mimics sepsis |
| Hematologic | Bleeding seen in only ~5% of ALF cases, but may increase with acute renal failure (ARF) and intracranial hypertension (ICH) |
| Renal | ARF can develop from acetaminophen toxicity, acute tubular necrosis, Wilson's disease, hepatorenal syndrome |
| Endocrine | Adrenal insufficiency should be considered if resuscitation and pressors do not improve hemodynamics; hypoglycemia can be seen in late disease |

- Several of the complications of ALF are listed in Table 9-9 and require active management in the ICU.
- Intubation and mechanical ventilation is necessary for patients with advanced encephalopathy (Grade III to IV), which this patient now has.

- Standing lactulose should be provided, although randomized controlled trials have not shown an improvement in outcomes with treatment. As the patient is now intubated, and for others who may be too somnolent to take this orally, an orogastric or nasogastric tube can be placed for administration. Alternatively, it can be provided via an enema.

- The leading causes of death from ALF are sepsis, which can lead to multi-organ system failure (MOSF), and cerebral edema leading to herniation, so careful monitoring and subsequent treatment of these are essential. Routine ICU management strategies are summarized in Table 9-10.

- Studies looking at the role of prophylactic antibiotics in ALF demonstrate a possible decreased incidence of infection but are inconclusive.

- Daily cultures and empiric antibiotics should strongly be considered in those with Grade III to IV encephalopathy, renal failure, or components of systemic inflammatory response syndrome, as infection is highly associated with these.

- With the progression of encephalopathy comes the increased risk for developing cerebral edema and intracranial hypertension (ICH).

- Routine insertion of an intracranial pressure (ICP) monitor is a debated issue and is typically center dependent. Monitoring may be reserved for those at high risk for cerebral edema or those awaiting orthotopic liver transplantation.

- Interventions are usually considered when ICP exceeds 20 to 25 mm Hg or cerebral perfusion pressure (CPP) declines to less than 50 mm Hg. This involves typical ICU maneuvers and treatments including proper body/head positioning, intravenous fluids, vasopressors, and correcting electrolyte abnormalities that can affect osmolality.

- Serum glucose levels may fall dangerously low in ALF, and close monitoring is essential with supplementation as needed—patients may require D10 infusions to maintain normal blood glucose levels.

**Table 9-10.**

## GOALS OF CARE IN THE INTENSIVE CARE UNIT

| | |
|---|---|
| HE | Standing lactulose, avoid sedatives, head computed tomography scan to exclude edema, hemorrhage, or mass lesion for advanced encephalopathy |
| Infection | Consider daily cultures, empiric antibiotics for high-risk ALF patients |
| Hemodynamics | Avoidance of hypotension with volume and pressors to achieve mean arterial pressure >75 mm Hg and CPP 60 to 80 mm Hg |
| Bleeding | Prophylaxis with proton pump inhibitor, consider trial of vitamin K, fresh frozen plasma/platelets only if indicated prior to invasive procedure |
| Renal failure | Volume resuscitation, avoidance of nephrotoxic agents, correction of associated electrolyte abnormalities, renal replacement therapy |
| Hypoglycemia | Continuous glucose infusion if persistent |
| Nutrition | Early initiation of enteral feeding, or parenteral if enteral not possible; protein restriction is not recommended |

*ICP monitoring has been initiated, and despite the above management, the patient's ICP remains elevated. What other treatment options should be considered for this worsening clinical course?*

- When the above options, along with other temporary measures such as mannitol, hypertonic saline, and increased sedation fail, additional novel modalities may be considered to bridge the patient to spontaneous recovery or possible transplantation.

- Therapeutic hypothermia (core body temp 32°C to 35°C) has been studied due to its effect of lowering ICP, revealing improvements in cerebral edema and ICH.[4]
  - Though the preliminary clinical studies are promising, additional randomized, controlled trials are necessary to confirm benefit and increased survival without causing significant harm before hypothermia becomes the standard of care for ALF-related cerebral edema.
  - Some of the potential unwanted outcomes at lower core body temperatures include the theoretical increased risk of infection due to alteration of immune function, cardiac dysrhythmias, and increased bleeding.
- Other treatment options being studied include plasmapheresis, drugs that facilitate ammonia excretion, and liver support devices such as bioartificial livers.[5] However, these therapies are experimental and are not part of standard treatment guidelines.

*Our patient remains intubated but has stabilized with reassuring hemodynamics and ICPs. What factors predict poor prognosis for transplant-free survival? What additional factors make him more or less likely to receive a transplant?*

- ALF due to acetaminophen overdose, hepatitis A, shock liver, or pregnancy is associated with higher transplant-free survival rates.
- There are several prognostic scores to help predict the outcome without liver transplantation, but there is no standard scoring system presently.
- The King's College Criteria (Table 9-11) is the most widely accepted and applied set of factors for predicting prognosis in ALF.
- Though the indices listed provide a good roadmap for the assessment of the patient's overall prognosis, the American Association for the Study of Liver

**Table 9-11.**

## KING'S COLLEGE CRITERIA FOR LIVER TRANSPLANTATION IN ACUTE LIVER FAILURE

| ACETAMINOPHEN-RELATED | NONACETAMINOPHEN-RELATED |
|---|---|
| Arterial pH <7.3 following resuscitation | PT >100 sec (INR >6.5) |
| *OR all of the following:* | *OR any 3 of the following:* |
| PT >100 sec (INR >6.5) *plus* | PT >50 sec (INR >3.5) |
| Serum creatinine >3.4 mg/dL *plus* | Drug-induced or indeterminate etiology |
| Grade III to IV HE | Jaundice to encephalopathy in >7 days<br>Age <10 years or >40 years<br>Serum bilirubin >17.5 mg/dL |

Diseases cautions against strict reliance of any available prognostic scoring system to predict outcomes and determine candidacy for liver transplantation.

- Cerebral hypoperfusion, with CPP less than 40 mm Hg for more than 2 hours, high-dose vasopressor requirements, and acute respiratory distress syndrome are some of the relative contraindications for transplantation.[6]
- According to the United Network for Organ Sharing, patients with ALF are given Status 1A priority when listed for orthotopic liver transplantation, higher than those with cirrhosis. The geographic area from where a liver originates is broadened, and waiting time is in the range of 2 to 4 days.

- The criteria for this listing include a life expectancy without transplantation less than 7 days; onset of HE within 8 weeks of symptoms; ICU-level care requiring either mechanical ventilation, renal dialysis, or severe coagulopathy (INR >2.0); and absence of pre-existing liver disease.[5]

- The 1-year survival rate for transplantation due to ALF is 58% to 92%, compared with 80% to 90% seen with chronic liver disease. The rate at 5 years is 61% to 76%.[7]

## Key Points

- ALF is characterized by coagulopathy and encephalopathy in a patient without previous liver disease.
- The most common identifiable etiologies in the United States are acetaminophen toxicity, nonacetaminophen drug reactions, and viral hepatitis.
- History taking should include ingestion of all prescription and nonprescription medications, herbal products, and dietary supplements, along with risk factors for viral hepatitis.
- Careful assessment of the clinical status is critical to determine if ICU level care is necessary; encephalopathic patients should be strongly considered for ICU admission given the rapidity of clinical decline.
- For confirmed or suspected acetaminophen-mediated ALF, immediate treatment with NAC is advised.
- Treatment of nonacetaminophen ALF with NAC in patients with early encephalopathy may improve transplant-free survival and should be strongly considered.
- Provide early treatment with acyclovir for suspected HSV- or VZV-related liver failure.
- In cases of ALF due to HBV infection, a nucleoside or nucleotide antiviral should be administered.
- Liver transplant service consultation should be done immediately in case rapid clinical deterioration occurs, requiring urgent evaluation or transfer to a transplant facility.

*(continued)*

---

### Key Points (continued)

- Infection associated with MOSF and cerebral edema leading to herniation are the leading causes of death related to ALF and should be aggressively sought after in the ICU.
- Know when to step up treatment for encephalopathy and ICH and when intubation with mechanical ventilation is needed.
- King's College Criteria provide a set of parameters to help predict prognosis in ALF and potentially direct toward liver transplantation.

---

# REFERENCES

1. Polson J, Lee WM. American Association for the Study of Liver Disease. AASLD position paper: the management of acute liver failure. *Hepatology*. 2005;41:1179-1197.
2. Lee WM, Hynan LS, Rossaro L, et al. Acute Liver Failure Study Group. Intravenous N-acetylcysteine improves transplant-free survival in early stage non-acetaminophen acute liver failure. *Gastroenterology*. 2009;137:856-886.
3. Tillmann HL, Hadem J, Leifeld L, et al. Safety and efficacy of lamivudine in patients with severe acute or fulminant hepatitis B, a multicenter experience. *J Viral Hepatol*. 2006;13:256-263.
4. Stravitz RT, Larsen FS. Therapeutic hypothermia for acute liver failure. *Crit Care Med*. 2009;37(7 suppl):S258-S264.
5. Stravitz RT, Kramer DJ. Management of acute liver failure. *Nat Rev Gastroenterol Hepatol*. 2009;6:542-553.
6. Torres DM, Stevens R, Gurakar A. Acute liver failure: a management challenge for the practicing gastroenterologist. *Gastroenterol Hepatol*. 2010;6(7):444-450.
7. Chan G, Taqi A, Marotta P, et al. Long-term outcomes of emergency liver transplantation for acute liver failure. *Liver Transpl*. 2009;15:1696-1702.

# 10

# Complications of Portal Hypertension

*Aarti Kakkar, MD*
*David P. Nunes, MD*

You receive the following call from an urgent care clinic:

*A 65-year-old man who recently emigrated from Vietnam presented to our office for his first physical. He reports a history of daily alcohol consumption, but stopped drinking alcohol several months ago. On exam: blood pressure (BP) 118/60, heart rate (HR) 72. He is anicteric with a normal abdominal exam, but you note gynecomastia. There are spider telangiectasias over his chest. Blood work shows the following results: platelets 110, international normalized ratio (INR) 1.20, aspartate aminotransferase (AST) 78, alanine transaminase (ALT) 53, alkaline phosphatase 98. Does this patient have portal hypertension (portal HTN)? What is the next step in evaluation?*

Lowe RC, Farraye FA.
*GI Emergencies: A Quick Reference Guide* (pp 167-188).
© 2012 Taylor & Francis Group

## WHAT IS PORTAL HYPERTENSION?

- Portal HTN refers to an elevation in portal venous BP, usually as a result of increased resistance to portal blood flow.
  - o This increase in outflow resistance can occur at the presinusoidal, sinusoidal, or postsinusoidal level.
- Portal HTN is defined by a portal BP of more than 12 mm Hg or a wedged hepatic venous pressure gradient (HVPG) of 5 mm Hg or more.
  - o Measurement of HVPG is a reliable indicator of portal HTN in sinusoidal causes of portal HTN (predominantly cirrhosis), but is less reliable in presinusoidal causes, which include portal vein thrombosis, schistosomiasis, etc. In pure presinusoidal portal HTN, the portal pressure is increased with normal HVPG.

## ETIOLOGY

- Cirrhosis is the most common etiology of portal HTN in the United States; however, portal HTN can also develop in patients without cirrhosis.
- Schistosomiasis is the most common cause of noncirrhotic portal HTN worldwide.
- Noncirrhotic causes of portal HTN can be divided into presinusoidal, sinusoidal, and postsinusoidal categories as shown in Table 10-1.

## DOES THIS PATIENT HAVE PORTAL HYPERTENSION?

### CLINICAL SIGNS AND SYMPTOMS

- This patient is from Southeast Asia, where hepatitis B is endemic, and he indicates longstanding alcohol

**Table 10-1.**

## CAUSES OF NONCIRRHOTIC PORTAL HYPERTENSION

| PRESINUSOIDAL* | SINUSOIDAL | POST-SINUSOIDAL |
|---|---|---|
| • Schistosomiasis<br>• Primary biliary cirrhosis<br>• Sclerosing cholangitis<br>• Sarcoidosis<br>• Congenital hepatic fibrosis<br>• Idiopathic portal HTN<br>• Portal vein thrombosis | • Arsenic poisoning<br>• Vinyl chloride toxicity<br>• Vitamin A toxicity<br>• Nodular regenerative hyperplasia<br>• Partial nodular transformation | • Veno-occlusive disease<br>• Budd-Chiari<br>• Right heart failure<br>• Constrictive pericarditis |

*In some causes of presinusoidal disease, the portal HTN may be mixed (ie, both pre- and sinusoidal; eg, schistosomiasis).

use—2 risk factors for developing cirrhosis. In addition, the presence of spider telangiectasias, thrombocytopenia, and elevated INR suggest a diagnosis of cirrhosis with portal HTN.

- Clinical symptoms, physical exam findings, and laboratory data that suggest portal HTN are listed in Table 10-2.

- The cirrhotic liver may be enlarged, normal, or small. However, the liver is usually hard or nodular in contour, and relative enlargement of the left lobe is an important clinical and radiological sign of cirrhosis.

- Loss of secondary sex characteristics, spider nevi, and palmar erythema are usually most marked in alcoholic cirrhosis.

**Table 10-2.**

## LABORATORY DATA THAT
## SUGGEST PORTAL HYPERTENSION

| CLINICAL SYMPTOMS | PHYSICAL EXAM | LABORATORY ABNORMALITIES |
|---|---|---|
| • Constitutional (fatigue, weight loss, anorexia)<br>• Easy bleeding or bruising<br>• Confusion<br>• Jaundice, dark urine<br>• Diarrhea<br>• Increased abdominal girth<br>• Lower extremity edema<br>• Pruritus | • Loss of secondary sex characteristics (testicular atrophy, gynecomastia)<br>• Fetor hepaticus<br>• Muehrcke's nails (paired horizontal white bands)<br>• Dupuytren's contracture<br>• Ascites<br>• Splenomegaly<br>• Asterixis<br>• Cruveilhier-Baumgarten murmur (venous hum over recanalized umbilical vein)<br>• Telangiectasias<br>• Palmar erythema | • Prolonged prothrombin time<br>• Thrombocytopenia<br>• Hypoalbuminemia<br>• Elevated globulins<br>• Decreased serum sodium<br>• Alkaline phosphatase elevated but less than 2 to 3x upper limit of normal (ULN)<br>• Hyperbilirubinemia<br>• Elevated liver function tests |

- AST and ALT are usually mildly elevated. In viral hepatitis, the AST/ALT ratio is normally less than 1, but with the development of cirrhosis, the AST/ALT ratio is often more than 1. The AST-to-platelet ratio index (APRI) (AST/ULN x 100/platelet count) is a simple noninvasive index of liver fibrosis (APRI >2.0 suggestive of cirrhosis).

## INITIAL EVALUATION

- The next step in evaluation would include a viral hepatitis panel and abdominal ultrasound to assess for features of cirrhosis and portal HTN, to assess the hepatic vasculature, and to exclude hepatic tumors.
- A liver biopsy remains the gold standard for identifying cirrhosis; however, clinical, radiographic, and laboratory data may obviate the need for liver biopsy.

## PATHOPHYSIOLOGY OF PORTAL HYPERTENSION

- The following morphologic and functional alterations in cirrhosis lead to the development of portal HTN:
  - Fixed obstruction to hepatic blood flow secondary to hepatic fibrosis and architectural changes.
  - Partially reversible presinusoidal obstruction via stellate cells, mediated by dysregulated endothelial nitric oxide synthases activity and nitric oxide production.
  - Intrahepatic vascular thromboses and vascular remodeling.
  - Increased portal venous inflow due to splanchnic vasodilation (Figure 10-1).

## COMPLICATIONS OF PORTAL HYPERTENSION

- Management of portal HTN entails addressing each of these complications as they arise (Table 10-3).

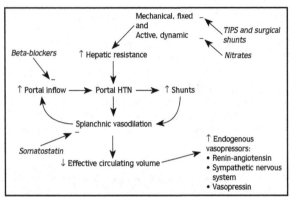

**Figure 10-1.** Pathophysiology of portal HTN. (Adapted from Laleman W, Van Landeghem L, Wilmer A, Fevery J, Nevens F. Portal hypertension: from pathophysiology to clinical practice. *Liver International.* 2005;25:1079-1090.)

**Table 10-3.**

## COMPLICATIONS OF PORTAL HYPERTENSION

| COMPLICATION | DEFINITION |
|---|---|
| Varices | Blood vessels in the esophagus, stomach, and rectum that dilate to decompress the hypertensive portal vein and are prone to bleeding (see Chapter 2). |
| Ascites/hepatic hydrothorax | Extra-cellular lymph within the peritoneal cavity. Hepatic hydrothorax results from accumulation of ascitic fluid in the pleural space. See next section. |
| Hepatorenal syndrome (HRS) | Renal failure in cirrhotics with refractory ascites due to extreme renal arterial vasoconstriction. See next section. |

*(continued)*

**Table 10-3.** *(continued)*

## COMPLICATIONS OF PORTAL HYPERTENSION

| COMPLICATION | DEFINITION |
| --- | --- |
| Hepatic encephalopathy | Neuropsychiatric disorder in cirrhotics due to portosystemic shunting and hepatocellular insufficiency. Treatment is aimed at discerning and addressing the precipitating event. Lactulose and rifaximin can be used to decrease gut ammonia production. |
| Hepatopulmonary syndrome | Dyspnea and hypoxemia due to intrapulmonary arteriovenous shunting mediated by endothelins. Diagnosed with contrast echocardiogram with agitated saline. Treatment is supplemental $O_2$ and liver transplant. |
| Portopulmonary syndrome | Vasoactive substances and shear stress with the pulmonary vasculature leads to increases in intrapulmonary vasoconstrictors and eventual obliteration of pulmonary arterioles. Cardiac catheterization reveals elevated pulmonary artery pressure (PAP) and pulmonary vascular resistance with normal pulmonary capillary wedge pressure. A mean PAP more than 35 mm Hg is a contraindication to liver transplant. Treatment: prostacyclin analogues, phosphodiesterase inhibitors, endothelin antagonists. |
| Neuroendocrine abnormalities | Arterial underfilling of sensory vascular beds leads to activation of the sympathetic nervous system, the renin-angiotensin-aldosterone axis, and increased antidiuretic hormone, resulting in fluid retention and reduced glomerular filtration rate (GFR). |

# Ascites

*A year has passed since you diagnosed hepatitis B and alcohol-induced cirrhosis in the patient presented at the beginning of this chapter. He presents to your office complaining of increased abdominal girth and lower extremity edema for the past several months. Abdominal exam reveals bulging flanks and shifting dullness. He has pitting edema. What is the next step in evaluation and treatment?*

## Development

- Three pathophysiologic processes contribute to the development of ascites:
    - Decreased intravascular oncotic pressure.
    - Sinusoidal portal HTN.
    - Activation of sodium and water retention due to perceived intravascular under-filling as a result of decreased systemic vascular resistance.
- The development of ascites in cirrhotic patients portends a 50% mortality rate within 3 years.[1]

## Evaluation and Diagnosis

### History and Physical Exam

- Eighty-five percent of patients with ascites will have cirrhosis.
- Nonportal hypertensive causes of ascites must be considered.
    - Intra-abdominal malignancy, kidney disease (most commonly nephrotic syndrome), heart failure, constrictive pericarditis, connective tissue diseases, pancreatic ascites, and a history of tuberculosis or asbestos exposure may be relevant.

- Physical exam findings include the following:
  - Shifting dullness has an 83% sensitivity and 56% specificity for detecting ascites. Approximately 1500 mL of fluid is needed to detect shifting dullness.[2]
  - A fluid wave, present in patients with large volume ascites.
  - Puddle sign (periumbilical dullness with the patient on his or her hands and knees) is said to be sensitive but may not be reliable.
  - Care should also be taken to assess the patient's overall fluid status by examining for lower extremity edema and jugular venous distension.

## Imaging

- An abdominal ultrasound with Doppler study should be performed at initial evaluation to assess for liver disease, hepatocellular carcinoma, and patency of the hepatic and portal veins. Ultrasound is also an accurate modality for detecting ascites if the physical exam is equivocal.

## Abdominal Paracentesis

- Abdominal paracentesis for fluid analysis is recommended in all patients presenting with new ascites.
- Paracentesis should be performed over an area of dullness to percussion.
  - The left lower quadrant, 2 finger breadths cephalad and 2 finger breadths medial to the anterior superior iliac spine, is usually the ideal place for needle insertion.
  - The midline, halfway between the pubis and umbilicus, and the right lower quadrant are also acceptable sites for needle insertion. The patient should empty his or her bladder prior to midline paracentesis to avoid bladder trauma.

- Complications of paracentesis are rare, but include abdominal wall hematoma (1%) and hemoperitoneum or bowel perforation (<1/1000).
- Because the bleeding risk is low, prophylactic use of fresh frozen plasma or platelets prior to paracentesis is not usually necessary even in the setting of a coagulopathy or moderate thrombocytopenia.
  - Concomitant renal failure increases bleeding risk.[3]

## FLUID ANALYSIS

- The purpose of performing a diagnostic paracentesis is 2-fold:
  - Determine the etiology of ascites, primarily whether it is due to portal HTN.
  - Assess for infection.
- Ascitic fluid analysis includes the following:

| Routine | Optional |
|---|---|
| Cell count and differential | Lactate dehydrogenase |
| Albumin | Amylase |
| Culture | AFB smear and culture |
| Gram stain | Cytology |
|  | Bilirubin |
|  | Triglyceride |

- pH, lactate, cholesterol, fibronectin, and glycosaminoglycans are not helpful.
- Serum albumin to ascites gradient (SAAG) obtained on same day—ascitic fluid albumin.
  - SAAG has replaced the transudate/exudate concept in classifying ascites.[4]
  - If SAAG is 1.1 g/dL or more, then the patient has portal HTN with 97% accuracy.

- o Approximately 5% of patients will have ascites due to more than one cause. In these patients, a SAAG of 1.1 or more still indicates that portal HTN is playing a part.
- o Spontaneous bacterial peritonitis (SBP) is defined by an absolute ascitic fluid polymorphonuclear (PMN) count of 250 cells/mm$^3$ or more (see SBP section on p. 181).
- o The gross appearance of the fluid is also helpful.
  - Uncomplicated ascites due to cirrhosis is yellow and translucent.
  - Cloudy fluid may indicate infection.
  - Pink or bloody fluid may indicate a traumatic tap, hepatocellular carcinoma, or malignancy-related ascites.
  - Milky or "chylous" ascites occurs when the fluid has a triglyceride concentration 200 mg/dL or more due to the presence of thoracic or intestinal lymph in the abdominal cavity.

| High Gradient Ascites, SAAG ≥ 1.1 | Low Gradient Ascites, SAAG < 1.1 |
|---|---|
| Cirrhosis | Peritoneal carcinomatosis |
| Alcoholic hepatitis | Peritoneal tuberculosis |
| Heart failure | Pancreatitis |
| Hepatic metastases | Serositis |
| Constrictive pericarditis | Nephrotic syndrome |
| Budd-Chiari | |

## TREATMENT OF ASCITES

- Patients with ascites due to portal HTN (SAAG ≥ 1.1) will respond to salt restriction and diuretics, whereas those with SAAG of less than 1.1 generally do not respond well to these measures, and the measures may be harmful.

- Management of ascites in patients without portal HTN is focused on addressing the underlying disease.

*Treatment of Noncomplicated Ascites*

**Diuretics/Sodium Balance**

- Low-sodium diet: 1500 to 2000 mg salt/day. More severe restriction is not well-tolerated and may have negative nutritional effects.
- The diuretics of choice for treating ascites are spironolactone and furosemide.
  - Furosemide inhibits sodium reabsorption at the loop of Henle. Care to avoid excessive diuresis and triggering pre-renal renal failure should also be taken when prescribing furosemide.
  - Spironolactone blocks mineralocorticoid receptors in the distal tubule, which antagonizes the hyperaldosteronemia of cirrhosis.
- Mild ascites may be initially treated with spironolactone alone.
  - Rapid natriuresis and maintenance of normokalemia can best be achieved with spironolactone 100 mg daily and furosemide 40 mg daily.
- If weight loss is inadequate, diuretics may be up-titrated every 3 to 5 days to a maximum dose of 400 mg spironolactone and 120 to 160 mg furosemide.
- Once lower extremity edema has resolved, expect approximately 0.5 kg/day of weight loss.[5]
- Amiloride can be substituted for spironolactone if tender gynecomastia develops but is generally less effective.
- The goal of sodium restriction and diuretics is to achieve a urinary sodium excretion of more than 78 mmol/day, resulting in a net loss of sodium and water. High sodium excretion without loss of ascites or weight strongly suggests noncompliance with sodium restriction.

      ○ A spot urine sodium that is greater than a spot urine potassium can indicate this with 90% accuracy.[4]

- Nonsteroidal anti-inflammatory drugs (NSAIDs) enhance sodium retention and are associated with treatment resistance and renal failure.
- Diuretics should be stopped and second-line options should be considered when there is uncontrolled encephalopathy, serum Na less than 120 mmol/L or serum Cr more than 2 mg/dL.

**Hyponatremia**

- Elevated antidiuretic hormone leads to impaired renal excretion of water and hyponatremia.
- Fluid restriction (1000 mL/day) should only be imposed on patients with dilutional hyponatremia (Na less than 120 to 125 mmol/L).
- Symptoms from hyponatremia do not typically develop until the serum Na is less than 110 mmol/L.[6]
- The place of vasopressin-2 receptor antagonists, "vaptans," in the management of hyponatremia and ascites is not yet defined, but may facilitate correction of hyponatremia and diuresis.

### Treatment of Refractory Ascites

*Your patient was diagnosed with high-gradient ascites due to portal HTN and cirrhosis. His ascites initially responded to a low-salt diet and 100 mg of spironolactone and 40 mg of furosemide. It has been 3 years since he developed ascites, and he has required up-titration to 400 mg spironolactone and 100 mg of furosemide. He is finally admitted to the hospital due to progressive abdominal distension and orthopnea. Exam is remarkable for BP 94/60, HR 55, tense ascites, scleral icterus, lack of lower extremity edema, and no asterixis. His lungs are clear, and a chest x-ray (CXR) is also negative. Labs are remarkable for an Na of 133, K 4.2, and Cr 1.0. You are consulted to aid in management of his ascites.*

- Ten percent of patients with ascites become refractory to medical therapy.[5]
- Initial evaluation for progressive ascites that was previously well-managed should include imaging to evaluate for a portal vein thrombosis and development of a hepatocellular carcinoma.
- A spot urine for sodium and potassium should be sent to assess for adequate sodium extraction and to detect noncompliance with a low-salt diet.
- Ascites that persists despite high-dose diuretics, or is complicated by encephalopathy, hyponatremia, hypokalemia, or azotemia, is defined as refractory.
- Repeated large volume paracentesis (LVP) and transjugular intrahepatic portosystemic shunts (TIPS) are available therapeutic options for this patient.[3]
- Several meta-analyses have shown that TIPS results in more effective control of ascites with more severe encephalopathy.[7-10]
- Randomized controlled trials have not definitively demonstrated improved survival or quality of life after TIPS (Table 10-4).[5,11]
- The preferred choice in managing refractory ascites is periodic LVP with plasma expanders if more than 5 L of fluid is removed.
  - Postparacentesis circulatory dysfunction: LVP results in activation of the renin-angiotensin and sympathetic nervous systems causing hypovolemia, hyponatremia, and azotemia.
  - Administering 8 g of albumin/L of fluid removed over 5 L has been shown to prevent postparacentesis circulatory dysfunction.[3,12]
  - Note: The yield from routine surveillance cell count and/or culture for large-volume peritonitis is very low (<5%) and is probably not indicated.
- Peritoneovenous shunts have been abandoned due to excessive complications, including infection, shunt occlusion, disseminated intravascular coagulation, and lack of survival advantage.

**Table 10-4.**

## CONTRAINDICATIONS AND DISADVANTAGES OF TRANSJUGULAR INTRAHEPATIC PORTOSYSTEMIC SHUNTS

| CONTRAINDICATIONS | DISADVANTAGES |
|---|---|
| Bilirubin >3 to 5 mg/dL | No improvement in mortality |
| Prothrombin time >20 seconds | No improvement in quality of life |
| Creatinine >2 mg/dL | TIPS stenosis |
| Model for End-Stage Liver Disease >18 to 20 | Liver ischemia/failure |
| Recurrent encephalopathy | Encephalopathy |
| Pulmonary HTN | Congestive heart failure |

- Patients with refractory ascites should be considered for liver transplantation.[3]

### Spontaneous Bacterial Peritonitis

*It is 3 months after your patient developed refractory ascites, which you elected to treat with serial LVP, when he is brought in by ambulance after being found lethargic and disoriented at home. History from the patient is limited, but he is alert to stimulation and can tell you his name. Exam is remarkable for T 98.1, HR 74, BP 99/55. His abdomen is distended with a fluid wave, and he is jaundiced. Neurologic exam is remarkable for asterixis. Routine blood work such as complete blood count, basic metabolic panel, and liver function tests are pending. CXR and urine analysis are clear. What is the next step in evaluation?*

- Abdominal pain, fever, encephalopathy, ileus, renal failure, acidosis, or leukocytosis can indicate SBP; however, given its high prevalence and mortality if left untreated, all hospitalized patients with ascites should undergo paracentesis to evaluate for SBP.[3]

- The prevalence of SBP in hospitalized patients with ascites is 10% to 30%.[13]

- SBP is thought to result from the translocation of bacteria from the intestinal lumen to lymph nodes causing bacteremia and infection of the peritoneal space. This is in contrast to secondary bacterial peritonitis, which is caused by a surgically treatable intra-abdominal process.

- SBP is defined by an ascitic fluid PMN count of 250 cells/m$^3$ or more.

- Fluid analysis must include a cell count with differential, gram stain, and culture. It has been shown that inoculation of the ascetic fluid directly into blood culture bottles increases the number of positive cultures by 20% or more. If secondary bacterial peritonitis is suspected, then ascitic total protein, lactate dehydrogenase, and glucose should be sent.

- Broad-spectrum, empiric treatment usually with a third-generation cephalosporin is the treatment of choice for SBP. Treatment should not be withheld until culture results return.[3] Aminoglycosides should be avoided.

- Outpatient management of stable patients without kidney dysfunction with oral antibiotics is appropriate.

- Successful treatment is marked by an improvement in clinical condition and a rapid reduction in fluid PMNs. A reduction of 25% to 50% within 48 hours of therapy should be seen. A failure to see a decrease in PMNs should initiate a reassessment of the antibiotic choice and a search for a secondary cause of peritonitis.

- If a polymicrobial infection is identified, a search for causes of secondary peritoneal infection is warranted.
- The following variants of SBP still warrant treatment:
  - Culture-negative neutrocytic ascites (PMNs ≥250, but culture-negative).
  - Mono-microbial non-neutrocytic ascites (PMNs <250, but culture-positive).

Besides prompt treatment with intravenous (IV) antibiotics, what other measures have been proven to improve survival in patients with cirrhosis and SBP?

- The hepatorenal syndrome (HRS) is the most severe complication of SBP and occurs in up to one-third of patients with SBP.
- Administration of albumin 1.5 g/kg of body weight on day 1 and 1.0 g/kg on day 3 of treatment prevents renal impairment and reduces mortality.[13]
- A more recent randomized trial indicates that patients with a Cr of more than 1 mg/dL, blood urea nitrogen (BUN) more than 30 mg/dL, or total bilirubin more than 4 mg/dL benefit the most from albumin administration; therefore, recent American Association for the Study of Liver Diseases guidelines recommend that only these patients receive albumin.[3,14]

*After 7 days of IV antibiotics and albumin on days 1 and 3 of treatment, the patient's encephalopathy has improved, Cr has remained stable, and there is no residual abdominal pain or fever. What is the next step?*

- There is a 70% probability of recurrence in 1 year after resolution of SBP.[5]
- Routine follow-up ascitic fluid analysis to document resolution of infection is not typically needed; exceptions include patients with persistent pain or fever and infection with atypical organisms.
- A previous episode of SBP warrants long-term, continuously dosed antibiotic prophylaxis, usually with a fluoroquinolone or trimethoprim/sulfamethoxazole

(TMP/SMX).[3] However, the later development of antibiotic-resistant infections remains a concern.

- Several randomized controlled trials revealed an improvement in mortality and reduction in bacterial infections in cirrhotics with risk factors for developing SBP (low protein ascites, variceal bleeding, and prior history of SBP) who were given antibiotic prophylaxis.[15-17]

# HEPATORENAL SYNDROME

*It is 1 month later, and your patient is readmitted with fever and encephalopathy. He has not been taking his prophylactic antibiotics regularly, and paracentesis confirms recurrent SBP. He receives IV albumin and antibiotics; however, his creatinine continues to rise. On hospital day 4, it is 3.0, and he is anuric. What is the diagnosis, and what treatment options are available?*

- One of the most serious complications of SBP is HRS, which is defined as a severe reduction in glomerular filtration rate (GFR) likely due to effective hypovolemia and renal vasoconstriction in the absence of significant renal histologic abnormalities.[5,18]
- Renal failure in cirrhosis may be caused by hypovolemia, NSAID use, intrinsic renal disease, or infection.
- Bacterial translocation, characteristic of SBP, is known to trigger production of pro-inflammatory cytokines and vasoactive mediators that affect circulatory function, worsen arterial under-filling, and cause intra-renal vasoconstriction.

## DIAGNOSIS

The diagnosis of HRS requires the following[18]:
- Cirrhosis with ascites
- Serum Cr more than 1.5 mg/dL

- No improvement of serum Cr after at least 2 days of diuretic withdrawal and volume expansion with albumin (1 g/kg a day)
- Absence of shock
- Absence of nephrotoxic drugs
- Absence of parenchymal renal disease

The HRS can be divided into Type I and Type II:

- Type I
  - Rapidly progressive renal failure, usually preceded by an inciting event
  - Doubling of initial serum Cr to a level more than 2.5 mg/dL in less than 2 weeks
  - Often associated with multi-organ dysfunction
- Type II
  - Slowly progressive and associated with refractory ascites
  - Moderate renal failure, Cr more than 1.5
- A diagnosis of HRS can only be entertained once the following evaluation has occurred:
  - Stop all nephrotoxic drugs and diuretics
  - Rule out structural abnormalities with ultrasound
  - Search for and treat underlying infection
  - A urinalysis with fewer than 50 red blood cells/high power field  and protein excretion less than 500 mg/day suggests absence of intrinsic renal disease
  - Urine sediment with renal tubular epithelial cells indicates acute tubular necrosis
  - Therapeutic trial of volume expansion with albumin

## TREATMENT OF HEPATORENAL SYNDROME

- The current approach to treating HRS focuses on volume expansion with albumin and vasoconstrictors.

- Current pharmacologic therapy in the United States consists of 1 g/kg of IV albumin plus the following:
  - Subcutaneous octreotide (a somatostatin analog) 200 mcg 3 times daily.
  - Oral midodrine (a selective alpha-1 adrenergic agonist) 3 times daily with a maximum dose of 12.5 mg/day to achieve an increase in mean BP by 15 mm Hg.
- Small, uncontrolled, nonrandomized clinical trials have shown a survival benefit and a reduction in serum Cr in patients treated with this regimen.[19]
- The vasopressin analog terlipressin reduces splanchnic vasodilation and increases GFR. It is used in Europe to treat HRS but is not currently approved for use in the United States.
- An alternative regimen is the use of noradrenaline, albumin, and furosemide.
- Liver transplantation is the only definitive treatment for HRS.
- Renal replacement therapy does not improve survival but can be used as a bridge to transplant or in those with acute, potentially reversible conditions such as alcoholic hepatitis.[5]

---

### Key Points

- In patients with liver disease, the presence of vascular spiders or thrombocytopenia are highly suggestive of portal HTN.
- Patients with ascites should undergo paracentesis at the time of diagnosis and when there is any sign of clinical deterioration. Initially, ascites should be sent for albumin, total protein, cell count (with differential), and culture. Calculation of the SAAG is essential in determining the etiology of ascites, and cell count/differential allows for rapid diagnosis of SBP.
- Up to 90% of patients with ascites respond to a combination of dietary sodium restriction and therapy with spironolactone and furosemide.    *(continued)*

---

## Key Points (continued)

- For patients with refractory large-volume ascites, LVP can be performed safely. If more than 5 L of ascites is extracted, infuse 8 g of IV albumin per liter removed to prevent hemodynamic and renal complications. In selected patients, TIPS can be effective in treating refractory ascites.
- Patients with SBP should be treated with a third-generation cephalosporin. Albumin infusion should be given on days 1 and 3 if patients meet the following criteria: serum BUN more than 30 mg/dL, creatinine more than 1 mg/dL, or bilirubin more than 4 mg/dL. After successful therapy of SBP, prophylaxis with a fluoroquinolone or TMP/SMX should be given.
- HRS should be considered in patients with cirrhosis and ascites who develop a rising creatinine, but a thorough evaluation must be undertaken to rule out other reversible causes of acute kidney injury. Patients diagnosed with HRS should be treated with midodrine, octreotide, and albumin.

# REFERENCES

1. Fernandez-Esparrach G, Sanchez-Fueyo A, Gines P, et al. A prognostic model for predicting survival in cirrhosis with ascites. *J Hepatol.* 2001;34:46-52.
2. Cattau EL Jr, Benjamin SB, Knuff TE, Castell DO. The accuracy of the physical exam in the diagnosis of suspected ascites. *JAMA.* 1982;247:1164-1166.
3. Runyon BA. Management of adult patients with ascites due to cirrhosis: an update. *Hepatology.* 2009;49(6):2087-2107.
4. Runyon BA, Montano AA, Akriviadis EA, Antillon MR, Irving MA, McHutchison JG. The serum-ascites albumin gradient is superior to the exudate-transudate concept in the differential diagnosis of ascites. *Ann Intern Med.* 1992;117:215-220.
5. Gines P, Cardenas A, Arroyo V, Rodes J. Management of cirrhosis and ascites. *N Engl J Med.* 2004;350:1646-1654.
6. Gines P, Berl T, Bernardi M, et al. Hyponatremia in cirrhosis: from pathogenesis to treatment. *Hepatology.* 1998;28:851-864.
7. Deltenre P, Mathurin P, Dharancy S, et al. Transjugular intrahepatic portosystemic shunt in refractory ascites: a meta-analysis. *Liver Int.* 2005;25:349-356.

8. Albillos A, Banares R, Gonzalez M, Catalina MV, Molinero LM. A meta-analysis of transjugular intrahepatic portosystemic shunt versus paracentesis for refractory ascites. *J Hepatol.* 2005;43:990-996.

9. D'Amico G, Luca A, Morabito A, Miraglia R, D'Amico M. Uncovered transjugular intrahepatic portosystemic shunt for refractory ascites: a meta-analysis. *Gastroenterology.* 2005;129:1282-1293.

10. Saab S, Nieto JM, Lewis SK, Runyon BA. TIPS versus paracentesis for cirrhotic patients with refractory ascites. *Cochrane Database Syst Rev.* 2006;4:CD004889.

11. Sanyal AJ, Genning C, Reddy KR, et al. The North American Study for the Treatment of Refractory Ascites. *Gastroenterology.* 2003;124:634-641.

12. Gines P, Tito L, Arroyo V, et al. Randomized study of therapeutic paracentesis with and without intravenous albumin in cirrhosis. *Gastroenterology.* 1988;94:1493-1502.

13. Sort P, Navasa M, Arroyo V, et al. Effect of intravenous albumin on renal impairment and mortality in patients with cirrhosis and spontaneous bacterial peritonitis. *N Engl J Med.* 1999;341:403-409.

14. Sigal SH, Stanca CM, Fernandez J, Arroyo V, Navasa M. Restricted use of albumin for spontaneous bacterial peritonitis. *Gut.* 2007;56:597-599.

15. Gines P, Rimola A, Planas R, et al. Norfloxacin prevents spontaneous bacterial peritonitis recurrence in cirrhosis: results of a double-blind, placebo-controlled trial. *Hepatology.* 1990;12:716-724.

16. Novella M, Sola R, Soriano G, et al. Continuous versus inpatient prophylaxis of the first episode of spontaneous bacterial peritonitis with norfloxacin. *Hepatology.* 1997;25:532-536.

17. Fernandez J, Navasa M, Planas R, et al. Primary prophylaxis of spontaneous bacterial peritonitis delays hepatorenal syndrome and improves survival in cirrhosis. *Gastroenterology.* 2007;133:818-824.

18. Salerno F, Gerbes A, Gines P, Wong F, Arroyo V. Diagnosis, prevention and treatment of the hepatorenal syndrome in cirrhosis: a consensus workshop of the international ascites club. *Gut.* 2007;56:1310-1318.

19. Angeli P, Volpin R, Gerunda G, et al. Reversal of Type 1 hepatorenal syndrome with the administration of midodrine and octreotide. *Hepatology.* 1999;29:1690-1697.

# 11

# Ischemic Disorders of the Gastrointestinal Tract

*Sujai Jalaj, MD*
*Daniel S. Mishkin, MD, CM, FRCP(C)*

You receive the following call from the emergency department:

*A 65-year-old man recently started on digoxin for atrial fibrillation awoke from sleep at 3 AM with severe periumbilical pain associated with diarrhea that later became bloody. The pain was knife like and severe enough that he knew he needed to seek medical attention immediately. The patient is sweaty and uncomfortable with an irregular heart rate of 100 beats per minute, complaining of generalized abdominal pain. His abdomen is tender but without peritoneal findings.*

The fear of vascular emergencies is due to the fact that time is of the essence as a lack of blood flow can lead to intestinal ischemia and subsequent gangrene. To improve clinical outcomes, an appropriate clinical suspicion and knowledge of the vascular anatomy supplying the gastrointestinal (GI) tract will help to provide a better understanding and differentiation of the various presentations associated with these events. Therefore, this chapter will review the vascular anatomy of the mesenteric

Lowe RC, Farraye FA.
*GI Emergencies: A Quick Reference Guide* (pp 189-208).
© 2012 Taylor & Francis Group

circulation, the different types of life-threatening and non-imminently life-threatening vascular emergencies, as well as the diagnostic and therapeutic options that should be considered even before reaching the bedside.

# VASCULAR ANATOMY OF
# SPLANCHNIC CIRCULATION

Three major vessels supply almost all of the blood flow to the digestive tract: celiac axis (CA), superior mesenteric artery (SMA), and inferior mesenteric artery (IMA).[1]

- CA: Arises from anterior aorta and supplies blood flow to the stomach, portions of the duodenum, and pancreas. CA gives rise to 3 branches:
    - o Left gastric artery
    - o Common hepatic artery, which has 3 branches: gastroduodenal, right gastroepiploic, and superior pancreaticoduodenal arteries
    - o Splenic artery, which has 2 branches: pancreatic and left gastroepiploic arteries
- SMA: Originates from the anterior aorta and supplies blood flow to a portion of the pancreas and duodenum, jejunum, and ileum, as well as the ascending and transverse colon. Branches of SMA typically form a series of arcades, and, from these arcades, numerous straight vessels arise and enter the intestinal wall. There are 4 major branches of SMA:
    - o Inferior pancreaticoduodenal artery
    - o Middle colic artery
    - o Right colic artery
    - o Ileocolic artery
- IMA: Originates from the anterior infrarenal aorta and supplies blood flow to the colon from the splenic flexure to the rectum. Major branches of IMA include the following:

o Left colic artery
o Sigmoid branches
o Superior rectal artery

# PATHOPHYSIOLOGY OF MESENTERIC ISCHEMIA

- Hypoxia of ischemia and reperfusion injury are the main mechanisms of ischemic damage.[2]
- Hypoxia of ischemia: Insufficient delivery of oxygen and nutrients due to lack of mesenteric blood flow leads to vasoconstriction that further exacerbates ischemia.
- Reperfusion injury: Formation of reactive oxygen radicals due to compromised mesenteric blood flow damages intestinal cells. Combination of hypoxia and reperfusion injury can lead to necrotic, gangrenous bowel if the ischemic period is prolonged.

# MESENTERIC ISCHEMIA

- Classification
  o Acute versus chronic mesenteric ischemia: Acute mesenteric ischemia (AMI) is more common.[3]
  o Arterial versus venous mesenteric ischemia: Arterial origin of ischemia is more common.[3]
  o Mesenteric versus colonic ischemia: Colonic ischemia is more common.
- Acute versus chronic
  o In AMI, it is important to remember that intestinal viability is threatened, and, so, bowel infarct is a potential outcome.
  o In chronic mesenteric ischemia, the major issue is that blood flow is inadequate to support functional demands of the intestine.

# SPECIFIC TYPES OF
# ACUTE MESENTERIC ISCHEMIA

- Arterial etiologies of AMI
  - Superior mesenteric arterial embolism (SMAE): Of the 3 major blood vessels that supply the bowel (CA, SMA, IMA), the SMA is most prone to emboli from any source, such as atrial fibrillation and indwelling lines.[3]
  - Nonocclusive mesenteric ischemia (NOMI): This is caused by vasoconstriction in the setting of myocardial infarction (MI), acute congestive heart failure (CHF) exacerbation, sepsis, medications/drugs (digoxin, cocaine), or pressors (norepinephrine, high-dose dopamine, vasopressin) in patients with underlying atherosclerosis.
  - Superior mesenteric artery thrombus (SMAT): Classic history associated with SMAT includes self-limited postprandial pain in weeks to months preceding acute onset of severe abdominal pain.
  - Focal segmental ischemia—Defined as vascular occlusion to small segments of the small bowel due to either vasculitis, atheromatous emboli, strangulated hernias, or radiation therapy.
- Venous etiologies of AMI
  - Superior mesenteric venous thrombosis (SMVT): Usually due to hypercoagulable states, portal hypertension (cirrhosis, congestive splenomegaly), malignancy, inflammation (pancreatitis, peritonitis), pregnancy, trauma, or surgery.

# CLINICAL ASPECTS OF
# ACUTE MESENTERIC ISCHEMIA

- Important clinical/medical history points to think about when consulted about possible AMI. Diagnosis of AMI requires high index of suspicion.

- o Cardiac: Is there a history of long-standing CHF? Use of diuretics and/or digoxin? Cardiac arrhythmias? Recent MI? Current/recent hypotension?
  - o Drugs: Use of cocaine? Required/requiring pressors?
  - o Sepsis?
  - o Recent hemodialysis with volume removal?
  - o Hypercoagulable state: Pregnant? New medication such as oral contraceptive pill? Active malignancy? Inflammation (pancreatitis, peritonitis)? Trauma? Abdominal surgery?
  - o Vasculitis?
  - o Liver failure: Portal hypertension (can lead to chronic mesenteric vein thrombosis)?
  - o History of postprandial abdominal pain in weeks to months preceding acute onset of severe abdominal pain? If so, this scenario is most commonly associated with SMAT.
  - o Recent instrumentation or line placement?
- Presence of abdominal pain
  - o Classic presentation is sudden onset of abdominal pain out of proportion to abdominal tenderness on exam.
  - o Pain is present in 75% to 98% of patients with AMI.[2]
  - o A sudden onset of severe abdominal pain accompanied by rapid and often forceful bowel evacuation, especially in the setting of minimal or no abdominal signs on exam, strongly suggests acute arterial occlusion typically due to SMAE.
  - o A more indolent and less striking onset of pain is more consistent with SMVT.
- Absence of abdominal pain
  - o Unexplained abdominal distention or lower GI bleeding may be the only indications of AMI, specifically NOMI.

- o Stool contains occult blood in 75% of patients.[2]
- o Also suspect NOMI in patients who have survived cardiopulmonary resuscitation and who develop bacteremia and diarrhea without abdominal pain.
- Presence of physical exam findings
  - o Abdominal findings (ie, tenderness, rebound tenderness, guarding) are typically absent only during the early course of AMI.
  - o Abdominal findings are present after prolonged AMI and, if present, usually signify intestinal infarct.

## LABORATORY FINDINGS/ DIAGNOSTIC STUDIES

- Lab results
  - o Seventy-five percent of patients have leukocytosis (white blood cell count >15,000).[4]
  - o Bowel infarction can be associated with metabolic acidosis (elevated serum lactate), elevated amylase, and serum phosphate.[4]
  - o Be sure to send complete blood count (CBC), serum lactate, and amylase to evaluate for bowel infarction.
- Imaging studies
  - o The first imaging studies to be performed include abdominal plain film and/or contrast-enhanced computed tomography (CT). With increased availability of CT scans, most proceed directly to cross-sectional imaging.
  - o Later on, when infarction has occurred, abdominal plain film reveals formless loops of small bowel, ileus, or "thumbprinting," which simply represents bowel wall edema and is seen in approximately 30% of patients with mesenteric ischemia.[5]

○ A contrast-enhanced CT can point to a diagnosis of AMI if pneumatosis, a thickened bowel wall, and/or portal venous gas is present, but it cannot rule out pre-infarct ischemia.[6]

○ Duplex ultrasound (US) is useful in identifying portal and/or SMV thrombosis and occasionally in identifying SMA thrombosis, especially if CT with contrast is contraindicated due to renal insufficiency, but it is not the first-line study of choice.

○ Contrast-enhanced CT is the diagnostic study of choice to detect SMVT.[7]

○ Cross-sectional imaging can be negative early in AMI, and clinical correlation is necessary.

○ Selective mesenteric angiography is the mainstay of diagnosis and initial treatment.

## DIAGNOSIS AND TREATMENT
## OF ACUTE MESENTERIC ISCHEMIA

*Adapted from guidelines proposed by the American Gastroenterological Association.[8]

- Diagnosis[8]
  ○ Selective mesenteric angiography is the diagnostic study of choice for both occlusive and NOMI, but it is not the first test to be performed.
  ○ CT of the abdomen is the diagnostic study of choice for SMVT, although mesenteric angiography can also be used and is more sensitive than CT.

- Treatment[8]
  ○ The initial step should involve volume resuscitation and discontinuation of pressors.
  ○ If pressors are required, dobutamine, low-dose dopamine, or milrinone are preferred because they have less of an effect on mesenteric perfusion.

- o Secondly, broad-spectrum antibiotics that cover both gram-positive and gram-negative organisms along with anaerobes should be started.
  - Broad-spectrum antibiotics have been shown to reduce the extent and severity of injury in experimental animals.
- o After addressing volume resuscitation, obtain cross-sectional imaging such as CT or magnetic resonance imaging (MRI) to rule out other causes of acute abdominal pain (ie, perforated viscus).
- o Imaging should be performed to rule out other causes of abdominal pain, rather than to rule in ischemia. If no alternative diagnosis is made, selective mesenteric angiography should be performed for diagnostic and possible therapeutic medication options.
- o During angiography, intra-arterial papaverine (vasodilator) can be infused because arterial vasoconstriction is the basis of NOMI and a contributing factor in all other forms of AMI.
- o Intra-arterial papaverine should be considered in all cases of AMI even if surgery is indicated/planned.
- o Regardless of what type of AMI is found, surgery is always indicated if there is evidence of necrotic/infarcted bowel, which is clinically suggested by peritoneal signs or on imaging studies.
- o Anticoagulation in management of AMI is controversial.
- o Anticoagulation with heparin infusion should be administered in cases of SMVT, SMAE, and SMAT.
- o If surgery is performed for AMI due to thrombus or embolus, anticoagulation should be started 48 hours postoperatively.
- o If diagnosis is not made before intestinal infarction, the mortality rate is 70% to 90%.[5,8]

○ Early diagnosis and treatment yields the best chances of survival, with a 90% survival in patients who had AMI, had no signs of peritonitis, and had angiography early in their course.

# FEATURES OF SPECIFIC TYPES OF ACUTE MESENTERIC ISCHEMIA

- SMAE
  - ○ SMAEs are typically differentiated from other forms of occlusive AMI based on location of the embolus.
  - ○ Angiography reveals a rounded filling defect with nearly complete obstruction to flow.
  - ○ SMAEs are further classified into "major" versus "minor" emboli.
  - ○ Emboli that lodge proximally to the origin of the ileocolic artery are considered "major" emboli, and clinically are more severe because they limit the collateral circulation.
  - ○ "Minor" emboli are emboli that lodge distally to the origin of the ileocolic artery.
- NOMI
  - ○ Usually results from splanchnic vasoconstriction caused by a preceding cardiovascular event (hypotension, acute hypovolemia, acute CHF, cardiac arrhythmias).
  - ○ If surgery is not indicated, treatment with papaverine infusion should be considered while attempting to correct the underlying etiology.
- SMAT
  - ○ Occurs in areas of severe atherosclerotic narrowing—most often at origin of SMA.
  - ○ Acute ischemic episode is usually superimposed on the chronic mesenteric ischemia—20% to 50% of patients with SMAT have a history of several weeks to months of postprandial abdominal pain, malabsorption, and weight loss.

- On angiography, it is difficult to distinguish between acute thrombosis and long-standing chronic SMA occlusion.
  - Typically, chronic SMA occlusion can be distinguished on angiography if prominent collaterals form between SMA and IMA and/or CA circulation.
  - Also, if there is good filling of SMA collaterals on angiography, occlusion is considered to be chronic.
- In summary, absence of collateral blood vessels or presence of collaterals with inadequate filling of SMA indicates an acute occlusion.

# SUPERIOR MESENTERIC VENOUS THROMBOSIS

- See p. 192 on Specific Types of AMI, which lists many of the predisposing conditions that cause SMVT.
- Clinical feature of SMVT can have acute, subacute, or chronic onset:
  - Acute SMVT: Clinically similar to presentation of acute arterial ischemia.
  - Subacute SMVT: Abdominal pain for weeks or months without evidence of bowel infarction.
  - Chronic SMVT: No history of abdominal pain but develop GI bleeding from varices; most patients bleed from gastroesophageal varices secondary to thrombosis and extension to present in a similar manner as portal hypertension.
- Duplex US, CT angiogram, and MRI have all been used to demonstrate SMVT.
- CT can diagnose SMVT in more than 90% of patients, so contrast-enhanced CT is the diagnostic study of choice.[6]
- When SMVT is diagnosed on CT, angiography is of limited value.

- When a history of deep vein thrombosis or a family history of an inherited coagulation defect is known in the setting of suspected AMI, contrast-enhanced CT is indicated as first imaging study.
- Because chronic SMVT presents with upper GI bleed, diagnostic evaluation of chronic SMVT is aimed at determining the cause of bleeding—upper endoscopy and abdominal imaging.
- If there are no signs of bowel infarction, acute/sub-acute SMVT can be treated with anticoagulation.

# CHRONIC MESENTERIC ISCHEMIA

- Definition: Recurrent episodes of non–life-threatening intestinal ischemia that are usually associated with eating.
- Pathophysiology: Recurrent abdominal pain is secondary to increased demand for gastric blood flow as food enters the stomach, a demand that is satisfied by "stealing" flow from small intestine.
- Risk factors: History of smoking and atherosclerosis (ie, coronary artery disease, peripheral vascular disease).
- Clinical manifestations: Symptoms worsen when demand increases (typically after meals).
    o Postprandial colicky abdominal pain, classically 30 minutes after eating and lasts a few hours.
    o Recurrent abdominal pain leading to food aversion and weight loss.
    o History of sitophobia (fear of eating due to anticipated abdominal pain) is highly suggestive of diagnosis.
    o In elderly patients, differential includes malignancy, pancreatitis, peptic ulcer disease, or chronic cholecystitis.
    o Physical exam may reveal abdominal bruit.

- Diagnosis
    - CT or MRI with intravenous contrast is the first diagnostic test.[9]
    - Demonstration of near or complete occlusion of at least 2 of 3 mesenteric vessels on imaging supports diagnosis.
    - Definitive diagnosis: Mesenteric angiography.[9]
    - If not technically limited, negative Doppler US has high negative predictive value, but a positive test should be followed by angiography.
- Treatment
    - Bypass surgery or percutaneous angiography with stenting should be performed to correct the limited blood flow. Increasing experience has been gained with stenting and is the procedure of choice because it is less invasive.

# COLONIC ISCHEMIA

- Background
    - Distinct clinical syndrome from mesenteric ischemia.
    - Primarily occurs in the elderly with evidence of atherosclerotic disease (ie, coronary artery disease, peripheral vascular disease).
- Pathophysiology
    - Nonocclusive disease secondary to alterations in systemic circulation or anatomic or functional changes in the local mesenteric vasculature.
    - No specific causes/triggers are typically identified.
    - "Watershed" areas, which include the splenic flexure and recto-sigmoid junction, are most susceptible to ischemia.
    - Most common ischemic bowel syndrome and is more common than mesenteric ischemia.[10]

- Risk factors[11]
  - Obstruction: Malignant mass, embolus, vascular obstruction related to arteritis.
  - Iatrogenic: Surgical procedures, aortic surgery.
  - Shock: Septic, cardiogenic, hypovolemic.
  - Drugs: Cocaine, amphetamines, digoxin, estrogen, danazol, vasopressin, psychotropic drugs, and gold compounds.
- Clinical manifestations
  - Most common symptom is cramping left lower quadrant pain with positive fecal occult blood test.
  - Urgent desire to defecate.
  - Bright red/maroon blood mixed with stool.
  - Fever and peritoneal signs should prompt suspicion for bowel infarction.
  - Physical exam: Abdominal tenderness over involved segment of bowel.
- Diagnosis
  - Diagnosis rests on clinical presentation and corroborative tests.
  - Abdominal plain film may show "thumbprinting" caused by bowel wall edema.
  - Abdominal CT with contrast showing thickened edematous involved colon.
  - Colonoscopy with biopsy may provide histologic confirmation.
  - Colonoscopy may show hemorrhagic nodules representing submucosal bleeding or dusky mucosa, ulceration, and segmental or extensive changes involving only one wall of the colon such as the presence of the colon single-stripe sign, a single longitudinal ulcerated or inflamed colon strip on colonoscopy.
  - Air insufflation during colonoscopy should be gentle to prevent further compromise of mucosal blood flow.

- o Isolated ischemia involving the right colon portends worse outcome with a 5-fold need for surgery and a 2-fold mortality compared with those with ischemia involving other colon regions.[12]
- o An area of debate is the utility of searching for cardiac sources of embolization in patients with ischemic colitis. A recent study found that transthoracic echocardiography identified cardiac sources of embolism in 43% of ischemic colitis patients versus 23% of age- and gender-matched control subjects.[13]
- o Conditions mandating anticoagulation, such as atrial fibrillation or dilated cardiomyopathy, were identified in 32% of case patients. Conditions requiring anti-arrhythmic therapy were identified in 25% of case patients.[13]
- Treatment[8]
  - o Hemodynamic support (IV fluids).
  - o NPO (nothing by mouth; allow bowel rest).
  - o Broad-spectrum antibiotics should be administered if there is fever, abdominal tenderness and/or leukocytosis, or long segment of colonic involvement.
  - o Serial abdominal exams to rule out development of peritoneal findings.
  - o Development of peritoneal findings: Obtain surgical consult for possible resection of affected colonic segment, not vascular reconstruction.
- Prognosis
  - o In more than half the patients with colonic ischemia, the disease is reversible.
  - o Generally, symptoms of colonic ischemia resolve in 24 to 48 hours, and the colon heals in 1 to 2 weeks.
  - o Potential complications include gangrene and perforation, segmental colitis, stricture, or universal toxic colitis.

- As a general rule, nongangrenous colonic ischemia is associated with a low mortality (approximately 6%).[12]
- Gangrenous ischemia is associated with a mortality as high as 50% to 75% with surgical resection and is almost always fatal if treated conservatively.[12]
- Mortality is higher if right-sided colonic ischemia is present given the potential implications of SMA territory.

## RETURN TO THE VIGNETTE

Returning to our clinical vignette, several features about our patient are striking, including age older than 60 years, history of cardiac disease, recent initiation of digoxin, sudden onset of severe periumbilical abdominal pain accompanied by rapid bowel evacuation, especially in the setting of minimal abdominal signs on exam, which strongly suggests AMI and, more specifically, SMAE. Bloody diarrhea may occur in patients with SMAE, and it is usually seen after abdominal pain has been present for several hours. Once there is suspicion of mesenteric ischemia, the goal of initial therapy is to maintain adequate perfusion to the gut. Initial therapy includes aggressive volume resuscitation with IV fluids and broad-spectrum antibiotics that include coverage against anaerobes. All medications that contribute to mesenteric vasoconstriction, in particular digoxin and epinephrine, should be discontinued.

Reaching a diagnosis promptly in order to provide appropriate treatment is of vital importance because it may take as little as 6 hours from the time of onset of ischemia until infarction occurs. Because our patient presents without peritoneal signs, workup at this point should include CBC with differential, serum lactate, and amylase along with plain film of the abdomen and/or contrast-enhanced CT in order to rule out other causes of abdominal pain. If imaging is unrevealing for other etiologies of abdominal pain and/or is suggestive of mesenteric ischemia, the patient should proceed to mesenteric angiography, and surgery should be consulted. Surgery should always be consulted when the diagnosis of mesenteric ischemia is being considered. If our patient had presented with peritoneal signs or was noted to have free air on imaging, then immediate surgical exploration would be indicated.

Ultimately, vascular emergencies involving the small and large bowel require a high index of clinical suspicion especially in patients with known risk factors (such as atrial fibrillation, CHF, peripheral vascular disease, or a history of hypercoagulability). Prompt diagnosis is extremely crucial in order to avoid progression to catastrophic complications of bowel infarction.

---

### Key Points

- Acute ischemia refers to several different clinical syndromes—acute embolic and acute thrombotic disease are of sudden onset and are typically life-threatening emergencies. NOMI may be acute or subacute in presentation but is frequently severe. Colonic ischemia, the most common ischemic syndrome, is often self-limited and not life-threatening. When discussing ischemic bowel syndromes, it is important to be specific in order to have a proper understanding of the etiology and prognosis of these disorders and to communicate the urgency of the situation to surgical and radiology colleagues (Table 11-1).
- A high index of suspicion for AMI must be maintained, as diagnosis in the first 12 hours of symptoms is associated with a much better prognosis than diagnosis after 24 hours (30% to 50% versus 70% to 90% mortality, respectively).

(continued)

## *Key Points (continued)*

- Sudden onset of pain with a less impressive abdominal exam ("pain out of proportion to exam") should prompt suspicion of AMI (especially embolic or thrombotic disease), especially in patients with risk factors for cardiovascular disease.
  - Patients should be asked about symptoms of "intestinal angina," characterized by severe pain approximately 30 to 60 minutes after meals. This may indicate chronic mesenteric ischemia, and acute pain in this setting may indicate thrombosis at the origin of the SMA. The presence of sitophobia and weight loss point even more strongly to chronic mesenteric ischemia.
  - In cases of suspected AMI, an abdominal CT should be performed to rule out other causes of acute abdominal pain; if no other etiology is found, then an angiographic study (CT, MR, or catheter-based) should be performed to confirm the diagnosis.
  - MVT has a different set of risk factors than arterial disease: hypercoagulable states, portal hypertension, malignancy, inflammation (pancreatitis, peritonitis), pregnancy, trauma, or surgery. It may present with acute or subacute pain, but chronic MVT may present with upper GI bleeding from esophageal varices.
  - Colonic ischemia is the most common form of intestinal ischemia, usually due to low flow in the colonic vasculature. Ischemic colitis typically affects "watershed areas" of the colon (splenic flexure, sigmoid colon) and spares the rectum. Clinically, it is characterized by left lower quadrant pain and occult blood or frank blood in the stool. It is generally self-limited, but in severe cases it can progress to transmural infarction and perforation. Typical cases resolve over 1 to 3 days with supportive measure (hydration, antibiotics), and angiography is generally not indicated (see Table 11-1).

**Table 11-1.**

## DISTINGUISHING FEATURES OF ACUTE COLONIC AND MESENTERIC ISCHEMIA

| ACUTE COLONIC ISCHEMIA | ACUTE MESENTERIC ISCHEMIA |
| --- | --- |
| 90% of patients over age 60 | Age varies with etiology of ischemia |
| Acute precipitating cause is rare | Acute precipitating cause is typical |
| Patients do not appear severely ill | Patients appear severely ill |
| Mild abdominal pain, tenderness present | Pain is usually severe, tenderness is not prominent early |
| Rectal bleeding, bloody diarrhea typical | Bleeding uncommon until very late |
| Colonoscopy is procedure of choice | Angiography indicated |

Reprinted with permission from Greenwald DA, Brandt LJ. Colonic ischemia. *J Clin Gastroenterol.* 1998;27:122-128.

# REFERENCES

1. Rosenblum JD, Boyle CM, Schwartz LB. The mesenteric circulation. Anatomy and physiology. *Surg Clin North Am.* 1997;77:289-306.
2. Brandt LJ, Feuerstadt P. Intestinal ischemia. In: Feldman M, Friedman LS, Brandt LJ, eds. *Sleisenger and Fordtran's gastrointestinal and liver disease: pathophysiology/diagnosis/management.* 9th ed. Philadelphia, PA: Saunders/Elsevier; 2010:2027-2048.
3. Reinus JF, Brandt LJ, Boley SJ. Ischaemic disease of the bowel. *Gastroenterol Clin North Am.* 1990;19(2):319.
4. Glenister KM, Corke CF. Infarcted intestine: a diagnostic void. *ANZ J Surg.* 2004;74(4):260.

5. Boley SJ, Sprayregan S, Siegelman SS, Veith FJ. Initial results from an aggressive roentgenological and surgical approach to acute mesenteric ischemia. *Surgery.* 1977;82:848-855.

6. Lee R, Tung HKS, Tung PHM, Cheung SCW, Chan FL. CT in acute mesenteric ischaemia. *Clin Radiol.* 2003;58:279-287.

7. Acosta S, Alhadad A, Svensson P, Ekberg O. Epidemiology, risk and prognostic factors in mesenteric venous thrombosis. *Br J Surg.* 2008;95:1245-1251.

8. Brandt LJ, Boley SJ. AGA technical review on intestinal ischemia. *Gastroenterology.* 2000;118:954-968.

9. Moawad J, Gewertz BL. Chronic mesenteric ischemia. Clinical presentation and diagnosis. *Surg Clin North Am.* 1997;77:357-369.

10. Higgins PD, Davis KJ, Laine L. Systematic review: the epidemiology of ischaemic colitis. *Aliment Pharmacol Ther.* 2004;19:729-738.

11. Longstreth GF, Yao JF. Diseases and drugs that increase risk of acute large bowel ischemia. *Clin Gastroenterol Hepatol.* 2010;8:49-54.

12. Greenwald DA, Brandt LJ. Colonic ischemia. *J Clin Gastroenterol.* 1998;27:122-128.

13. Hourmand-Ollivier I, Bouin M, Saloux E, et al. Cardiac sources of embolism should be routinely screened in ischemic colitis. *Am J Gastroenterol.* 2003;98:1573-1577.

# 12

# Caustic Ingestions, Foreign Bodies, and Food Impactions

*Jennifer A. Sinclair, MD*
*Charles M. Bliss Jr., MD, FACP*

You receive the following call from the emergency department (ED):

> We have a 46-year-old male with a history of hypertension and asthma who came in with the feeling of "food getting stuck" when he swallowed. He was at a barbecue, ate a piece of steak, and when he swallowed, he felt it become "lodged in his chest." He tried to drink water to help it go down, but says he vomited the water. He is hemodynamically stable, and we are awaiting your advice.

## FOOD IMPACTIONS

Food impactions are a common gastrointestinal (GI) emergency. Both food impactions and foreign bodies tend to become lodged in the esophagus at different locations, depending on age of the patient. In children, impactions

Lowe RC, Farraye FA.
*GI Emergencies: A Quick Reference Guide* (pp 209-226).
© 2012 Taylor & Francis Group

typically occur at the level of the cricopharyngeus, which is the narrowest part of the esophagus for a child. In adults, they most frequently occur at the lower esophageal sphincter, where strictures or rings are more common, or occur at other sites of abnormal pathology.[1]

## WHAT IS THE TIMING AND NATURE OF THE INGESTION?

- Use the following information to determine the necessity and urgency of removing the item:
  - If symptoms suggest the bolus is impacted in the esophagus, it is likely that urgent endoscopy will be indicated.
  - Most esophageal food impactions will pass on their own, but a bolus remaining in the esophagus for a prolonged period of time increases the risk of esophageal ulceration and perforation, so the nature of the ingestion and timing become important factors in determining urgency.
  - If the patient is in significant distress or is having trouble managing their secretions, the procedure will need to be performed emergently. If not performed urgently, esophagogastroduodenoscopy (EGD) should certainly be performed within 24 hours.[2]
  - If EGD is indicated, the nature of the impaction will help determine what tools might be useful therapeutically.

## GET BACKGROUND INFORMATION ABOUT THE PATIENT TO HELP MINIMIZE THE RISKS OF THE PROCEDURE

- Although it is likely you will need to perform endoscopy to remove the bolus, you can still make a quick assessment of the safety of the procedure.
  - Can they physically tolerate the procedure?
    - Will their hemodynamics and volume status tolerate sedation? Or should they be given intravenous (IV) fluids prior to the procedure?

**Table 12-1.**

## THE AMERICAN SOCIETY OF ANESTHESIOLOGY RISK CLASSIFICATION

| ASA Class 1 | A normal healthy patient |
|---|---|
| ASA Class 2 | A patient with mild systemic disease |
| ASA Class 3 | A patient with severe systemic disease |
| ASA Class 4 | A patient with severe systemic disease that is a constant threat to life |
| ASA Class 5 | A moribund patient who is not expected to survive without the operation |

ASA *Physical Status Classification System.* 2009. http://www.
asahq.org/clinical/physicalstatus.htm is reprinted with permission
of the American Society of Anesthesiologists. A copy of the full text
can be obtained from ASA, 520 N. Northwest Highway, Park Ridge,
Illinois 60068-2573.

- What is the patient's risk of conscious sedation? The American Society of Anesthesiology (ASA) class should be determined before any endoscopic procedure (Table 12-1).[2]
- Will you need help with managing the airway? If the ASA class is greater than 3, the patient has increased risk of apnea (such as underlying obstructive sleep apnea or morbid obesity), or if the endoscopist anticipates a long, complicated procedure, you may consider an anesthesia consult for help managing the airway during the procedure.
- Do they have coagulopathy that would make a procedure risky and that should be reversed prior to a procedure?
    - Do they take anticoagulants?
    - Do they have underlying liver disease? Thrombocytopenia?

□ Do they need a blood transfusion? Vitamin K? Platelets?

## WHO WILL BE GIVING CONSENT? ASK THIS UP FRONT

- Most patients will provide their own consent, but in cases where the patient is accompanied by a family member to provide consent, there is a risk the family member will disappear prior to your arrival in the ED. Remembering that you can get consent over the phone with the emergency room (ER) physician as a witness can save the time of trying to track down a family member that just "went to wait outside."

*The patient reports the time of ingestion as 1 hour prior to coming to the ER. Blood pressure is 130/70, heart rate is 85, and he appears healthy except that he is spitting his saliva into a basin. The patient takes aspirin 81 mg daily, denies the use of blood thinners, has no known liver disease, and does not drink alcohol. He is alert and can provide his own consent. Based on hemodynamics and risk, he sounds appropriate for endoscopy, and because he is unable to swallow his secretions, the steak will need to be removed tonight. The ER resident asks if there is any testing you would like performed prior to your arrival.*

## OBTAINING LABS IS OPTIONAL

- Complete blood count (CBC) and international normalized ratio (INR) will not likely alter your plan to do endoscopy but may help assess the risk of bleeding complications and identify reversible abnormalities should bleeding occur.

## CONSIDER GLUCAGON

- Administer glucagon 1 mg IV. This should not delay an endoscopy but can be helpful in relaxing the esophagus to let the bolus pass. Ask the ED physician to administer glucagon while you are in transit to see the patient. Caution should be used in diabetics because glucagon can precipitate a rebound hypoglycemia. The effectiveness of glucagon is variable; in healthy subjects, it has been shown to reduce lower esophageal sphincter pressure effectively, but in impaction secondary to a fixed lesion such as a ring or stricture, it will be ineffective.

- Proteolytic enzymes like papain should *never* be used in a food impaction. It will increase the risk of esophageal perforation.[2,3]

## IMAGING IS NOT TYPICALLY INDICATED

- Imaging may be indicated if physical exam is suspicious for perforation, but if suspicion is low, a plain film is sufficient. Computed tomography (CT) is more sensitive for detection of microperforation, so if suspicion of perforation is higher, consider CT with oral gastrografin to look for esophageal leaks.

*You head into the ER to evaluate the patient. Upon arrival, you learn that the glucagon was ineffective. You perform a brief physical exam that notes lack of significant cardiac or pulmonary disease and no stigmata of portal hypertension. You plan for endoscopy to remove the steak with conscious sedation and call the attending to come in. You begin to prep for the procedure.*

- Obtain consent.
- Set up for the procedure.
  - Nursing questions:
    - Do you need to order medications for sedation? Conscious sedation typically requires anywhere from 50 to 125 mcg of fentanyl and 2 to 4 mg of midazolam (Versed). A large, tolerant person may need up to 150 mcg of fentanyl and 6 to 8 mg of Versed. Ask the nurse to draw up the maximum you think you will need.

- Will they set up 2 wall suctions (one airway, one for the scope)?
- Can they place the patient on oxygen for the procedure? A 2-L nasal cannula is sufficient.

  o Set up your equipment, making sure the foreign body supplies include the following[2,4]:

    - Hood: A bell-shaped rubber instrument that attaches to the end of the scope initially in an inverted orientation. After grasping a sharp foreign body in the stomach with forceps and starting to withdraw the scope, the hood will catch on the gastroesophageal (GE) junction and flip over the object, protecting the esophagus from further damage by the object.
    - Roth nets.
    - Snares.
    - Overtube (esophageal and gastric lengths): A plastic tube that can be introduced into the esophagus by endoscope and then kept in place to protect the oropharynx and esophagus from damage due to multiple passes of the endoscope into and out of the esophagus.
    - Rat-toothed forceps or alligator forceps and standard forceps.

- Write your note while you're waiting for the attending to arrive.

*You perform the EGD, finding a 2-cm bolus of steak impacted in the distal esophagus. You grasp it with the rat-toothed forceps and remove it piecemeal, protecting the esophagus and upper airway with a hood. Eventually, you are able to get the scope around it and confirm no distal blockage. You then push the remainder of the bolus into the stomach. The patient tolerates the procedure well and can recover from conscious sedation in the ER before returning home.*

> ### Key Points: Food Impactions
>
> - If a patient is in severe distress or is unable to swallow secretions, endoscopy must be done emergently. Otherwise, it can be postponed until a reasonably convenient time. After 24 hours, the complication risk increases, so it should be performed within the first 24 hours.
> - There is a high incidence of underlying esophageal pathology in patients with food impaction (eosinophilic esophagitis, Schatzki ring, peptic stricture, cancer). A bolus should not be pushed distally unless the scope can pass the bolus to evaluate the distal esophagus and exclude pathology first. If appropriate, the esophagus can be biopsied at the time of the procedure to exclude eosinophilic esophagitis. Otherwise, they should be scheduled to come back for an elective EGD.

# FOREIGN BODY INGESTION

*It's 6 PM on Friday evening, and you are just getting ready to sign out when you receive a page requesting you come to the ER to evaluate a 42-year-old patient who was eating appetizers at happy hour with his colleagues after work and swallowed a piece of chicken bone. He's complaining of constant, substernal pain that is sharp but is only causing mild discomfort.*

## WHAT WAS SWALLOWED AND WHEN?

- Objects that can lodge in the GI tract can be divided into 2 categories: blunt (buttons, coins, gastrostomy tube bumpers) and sharp (fish bones, toothpicks, dental hardware).[1,3] This will help guide your procedure.
- Urgency of endoscopy is determined by risk of perforation or aspiration. Emergent endoscopy will be required in 3 cases[1]:

o Sharp foreign body or disk battery
  ▪ The most dangerous sharp objects are chicken and fish bones, straightened paperclips, toothpicks, needles, and dental bridge work.
  ▪ Disk batteries may cause liquefaction necrosis in the esophagus through leakage of alkali and may generate electrical current that can be corrosive, but once past the esophagus, they typically pass through the rest of the GI tract without incident (85% in 72 hours).
o High-grade obstruction of the esophagus with inability to manage secretions
o Acute distress
- You should never attempt to retrieve narcotic packets—the risk of rupture is high. Surgical intervention is indicated for failure of the packets to progress, signs of obstruction, or suspected rupture.[2]

## Is It Safe to Perform the Procedure?

o It is likely that you will need to perform urgent endoscopy, but you can still optimize the patient prior to the procedure.
o Is he or she hemodynamically stable?
  ▪ Can he or she be sedated, particularly noting respiratory status? If you anticipate a long or difficult procedure, it may be helpful to electively intubate him or her for airway protection.
o Does he or she have a coagulopathy that you should start reversing?

*The patient is hemodynamically stable, and the physical exam is unremarkable. The ER staff asks if you would like them to do any further evaluations while you are on your way in.*

## Obtaining Labs Is Optional

- CBC and INR will not likely alter your plan to do endoscopy, but may help assess the risk of bleeding complications and identify reversible abnormalities should bleeding occur.

## Imaging Is Helpful, Particularly When Performed Within 1 Hour of Performing the Procedure

- Plain films may be helpful in locating the object because most foreign objects are radio-opaque.[2] The exceptions are objects such as fish bones, wood, plastic, and glass, in which case plain films are useful for excluding perforation but not localization.
    - Films should focus on the area where the patient has discomfort.
    - Contrast generally should not be administered for 2 reasons:
        - If the object is in the esophagus, contrast may be aspirated. Even gastrografin can cause a chemical pneumonitis.
        - Contrast coats the object and the mucosa, making visualization more difficult on endoscopy.
        - If symptoms really are not clear or specific, cautious use of contrast may be necessary, but if symptoms are esophageal and persistent, EGD should be performed despite a negative study.
    - If the object is small, films should be repeated within 1 hour of endoscopy to confirm the object is still in the esophagus or stomach.
    - Objects at or above the cricopharyngeus muscle should be removed by rigid endoscope or laryngoscope with forceps by enlisting otolaryngology or thoracic surgery. More distally, a flexible endoscope can be used.

*You head to the ER to evaluate the patient. He is a healthy-appearing man in mild distress. Because he has swallowed a sharp object, you decide to perform the EGD now, rather than waiting. You call your attending, and begin setting up for the procedure while waiting for the attending to arrive.*

- Obtain consent.
- Set up for the procedure.
  - Nursing issues:
    - You will need 2 suctions—one for the scope, one for the patient's airway.
    - Ask if they need you to order medications for sedation.
    - Ask them to place the patient on supplemental oxygen for the procedure.
  - Check your equipment. Equipment should include rat-tooth or alligator forceps, snares (helpful for coins), stone retrieval basket (helpful for smooth, round objects like marbles), overtube, hood, Roth net (for more details, see the prior section on equipment for food impactions).
- Write your note while waiting for the attending to arrive.

*You perform an upper endoscopy under conscious sedation and find a 2-cm long piece of chicken bone lodged just proximal to the GE junction at the level of a Schatzki ring. You are able to retrieve it using a snare with the hood to protect the esophagus, but don't have equipment to dilate the ring. You return the patient to the ED team for further management and instruct the patient to maintain a soft diet until he can have the ring dilated during regular hours.*

## *Key Points: Foreign Bodies*

- Determining urgency
  - ¤ Emergent endoscopy is indicated for sharp foreign bodies and esophageal button batteries. Smooth items smaller than 5 to 8 cm in length are likely to pass on their own and can be monitored with serial imaging.
  - ¤ Endoscopy is indicated within 24 hours for all esophageal foreign bodies (emergently if the patient is in severe distress or there is high-grade obstruction as evidenced by inability to manage secretions), but films should be obtained within 1 hour of the procedure to confirm the item is still in the esophagus.
  - ¤ Once an item enters the stomach, it is likely to pass within 72 hours through the entire GI tract, although this ranges from 3 to 6 days. If it is sharp, it should be removed from the stomach or duodenum as soon as possible. If it is larger than 5 to 8 cm in length, it is unlikely to pass the duodenal sweep and should be removed as soon as reasonably convenient.
- Imaging
  - ¤ Should be used to confirm location and exclude perforation.
  - ¤ Contrast should almost never be given.
- Technique
  - ¤ Airway should be protected at all times with the use of a hood, overtube, or intubation.
  - ¤ The risk of iatrogenic perforation can also be reduced by use of a hood or overtube, but the object should also be retrieved blunt-end first.
  - ¤ Anesthesia assistance with sedation is helpful for ASA class higher than 3 or if the procedure is anticipated to be particularly long or difficult.
  - ¤ Objects impacted in the esophagus should not be pushed down into the stomach until after the more distal esophagus has been examined because, frequently, underlying pathology has caused the impaction.
- Follow-up: When all else fails...
  - ¤ Most objects that pass the pylorus will pass the entire GI tract in 4 to 6 days but may take up to 4 weeks. Patients should be instructed to monitor their stools, and films should be obtained weekly to document progression. Surgery is indicated for objects that remain within the stomach after 3 to 4 weeks or that remain in the same location for more than 1 week.[3]

## CAUSTIC INGESTIONS

*A 35-year-old woman with a history of bipolar disorder is brought by her husband to the ED for lethargy. She is arousable, but not able to provide history, and her husband reports he returned from a short trip to the grocery store and found her sitting on the floor crying with a bottle of drain cleaner in her hand. She reported to him that she drank it in a suicidal gesture and complained of severe epigastric pain before becoming obtunded. The ED has sent basic labs and a toxicology screen, but the results are pending.*

### WHAT WAS INGESTED AND WHEN?

- The degree of mucosal injury depends on the acidity of the agent, the amount, the concentration, and the duration of exposure.[1,5]
  - Alkali agents cause rapid, penetrating liquefaction necrosis within seconds. Over months, this will progress to fibrosis. Alkali will damage esophagus and stomach and progress into the small bowel and are typically more viscous, causing longer contact time with the tissue.
  - Acidic agents cause superficial coagulation necrosis with scarring. This may limit the extent of injury. Acid will damage the stomach more than the esophagus.
  - Inflammation/ulceration: Bleeding, mediastinitis, peritonitis, shock, perforation, death.

### HAS IMAGING BEEN PERFORMED?

- Initial management of the patient will be supportive, but if there is a perforation, the patient will need emergent surgical evaluation rather than endoscopy.

*The ER resident tells you the patient is stable, with plans to admit to the intensive care unit (ICU). They discussed that the particular drain cleaner her husband found is composed of sodium hydroxide, with a pH of 13 to 14. Portable chest and abdominal plain films show no evidence of perforation, but the surgical consult is currently seeing the patient anyway. They ask if you will be coming to the ER to see the patient and if there are any other evaluations you would like in the interim.*

## Imaging Should Be Performed to Exclude Perforation

- Plain films may be sufficient, but if suspicion for a perforation is high, a gastrografin swallow with upright chest film or oral contrast with CT will increase the sensitivity of detecting a small perforation.[1,5]
- Surgery is indicated if there is perforation or if there is high clinical suspicion for perforation even in the setting of unrevealing films.
  - Physical exam should include checking the oropharynx for blistering or ulcerations and checking the neck for crepitus.

## Where Is the Patient Going to Be Admitted?

- Endoscopy is indicated in the first 12 to 24 hours after the injury in order to grade the injury and provide prognostic information. In the immediate management, the patient needs to be stabilized.[1,5]
  - Admission to the ICU is appropriate for aggressive volume resuscitation and support.
- A nasogastric tube should not be placed blindly because of the risk of perforation.
- The effect of acid suppression with a proton pump inhibitor (PPI) has not been studied, but PPI is typically administered simply because it is a reasonable intervention without adverse effects.

## Initial Management Should Consist Primarily of Observation

- Initial trials suggested reduced incidence of stricture formation with steroid administration in the acute setting, but subsequent prospective data have shown no therapeutic benefit to steroids.[5]
- Attempts at neutralization of acid were also not shown to be helpful and in fact may cause an exothermic reaction that results in worsening of the injury.
- Inducing emesis exposes the esophagus a second time to the caustic agent.
- Empiric antibiotics have not been shown to have any benefit.

*You agree with the plan to admit the patient to the ICU and recommend they keep the patient NPO (nothing by mouth). In the morning, you arrive early to ensure the patient is appropriate for an endoscopy. Her husband gives consent for the procedure, and you perform an EGD, noting severe esophagitis that involves 75% of the circumference of the lumen.*

## Grade the Mucosal Injury

- Long-term sequelae of caustic injury include esophageal or gastric antral strictures and increased risk of squamous cell cancer of the esophagus.
- The goal of endoscopy in caustic ingestion is to grade the injury (Table 12-2), rather than to provide an intervention because the degree of injury does correlate with the risk of long-term complications.[5]
- Table 12-2 provides valuable prognostic information:
  - Grade 0 and I injuries don't typically have long-term sequelae.
  - Grade II injuries have a 30% chance of developing strictures.
  - Grade III injuries have an 80% chance of developing short- and long-term strictures. These can present anywhere from 1 month to 1 year after the

**Table 12-2.**

## GRADING SYSTEM FOR MUCOSAL INJURY

| GRADE | ENDOSCOPIC FINDINGS |
|-------|---------------------|
| 0 | Normal esophagus |
| I | Superficial edema and erythema |
| II | Superficial ulcer |
| IIa | Superficial ulcer, erosion, exudate |
| IIb | Deep discrete ulcers or circumferential ulceration |
| III | Transmural ulceration with necrosis |
| IIIa | Focal necrosis |
| IIIb | Extensive necrosis |
| IV | Perforation |

ingestion. These patients should be hospitalized for the immediate supportive care and will need surveillance after the acute issues have resolved.

### ADVANCING DIET DEPENDS ON THE DEGREE OF INJURY

- Patients with Grade I through III injuries can be started on a liquid diet within 24 to 48 hours and advanced as tolerated.
- More severe injuries may require parenteral nutrition, which has been shown to improve outcomes.

### RECOMMEND APPROPRIATE MONITORING

- Patients with Grade II injuries should have close follow-up for development of dysphagia or gastric outlet obstruction, which may require serial dilations or resection.[5]

- Patients with Grade III injuries are at high risk of perforation and require close monitoring for at least 1 week.

## HELP SCHEDULE FOLLOW-UP

- Caustic ingestion increases the risk of eventually developing carcinoma at the area of esophageal scar (but not gastric cancer). Mean incidence occurs at 41 years after ingestion.
- The American Society for Gastrointestinal Endoscopy guidelines recommend surveillance endoscopy every 1 to 3 years beginning 15 to 20 years after the ingestion for early detection of esophageal carcinoma.[2]

---

### Key Points: Caustic Ingestions

- Alkali ingestions cause more damage than acidic, particularly to the esophagus. Initial management should focus on excluding perforation and aggressive supportive care. Resist the temptation to start antibiotics or steroids or to induce vomiting.
- The role of endoscopy in caustic ingestions is prognostic rather than therapeutic. EGD should be performed within 12 to 24 hours of ingestion to grade the injury.
  - ◻ Grade II patients may be discharged with outpatient follow-up.
  - ◻ Grade III patients should be hospitalized.
- There is no evidence to support steroids, antibiotics, or PPI in the initial management of caustic ingestion, although PPI is typically given because of the benign side-effect profile.
- Inducing emesis and attempting to neutralize the ingested substance are contraindicated.
- There is evidence for early nutritional support with parenteral nutrition in healing severe injuries.

# REFERENCES

1. Betalli P, Rossi A, Bini M, et al. Update on management of caustic and foreign body ingestion in children. *Diagn Ther Endosc.* 2009;2009:969868.
2. Eisen GM, Baron TH, Dominitz JA, et al; American Society for Gastrointestinal Endoscopy. Guideline for the management of ingested foreign bodies. *Gastrointest Endosc.* 2002;55(7):802-806.
3. Ginsberg GC. Management of ingested foreign objects and food bolus impactions. *Gastrointest Endosc.* 1995;41(1):33-38.
4. Smith MT, Wong RK. Foreign bodies. *Gastrointest Endosc Clin N Am.* 2007;17(2):361-382.
5. Lee M. Caustic ingestion and upper digestive tract injury. *Dig Dis Sci.* 2010;55:1547-1549.

# 13

# Complications of Endoscopy

*Jennifer A. Sinclair, MD*
*Caroline Loeser, MD*

You receive the following call from the emergency department (ED):

*We would like to discuss a patient known to your service who has presented with a fever. The patient was seen in endoscopy yesterday for an esophago-gastroduodenoscopy (EGD) with esophageal dilation. He regularly needs dilation for a benign stricture after a caustic ingestion as a child. As far as we know, the procedure was uncomplicated, and the patient was discharged home. The patient was doing well until this morning, when he started to feel short of breath and noted a fever. We are concerned that his symptoms are related to the procedure.*

Upper endoscopic diagnostic and therapeutic procedures carry a low risk of complications, estimated to be approximately 0.1%. Complications of upper endoscopy typically fall into one of several categories, including problems from sedation, cardiopulmonary complications, infection, bleeding, and perforation.

Lowe RC, Farraye FA.
*GI Emergencies: A Quick Reference Guide* (pp 227-258).
© 2012 Taylor & Francis Group

# In General

- Complications from sedation and cardiopulmonary events account for about 40% of all upper endoscopy complications and can be reduced by careful patient selection, consideration of patient comorbidities, and appropriate use of sedation, including involvement of an anesthesiologist if the procedure is anticipated to be long or complicated.

- Infection, bleeding, and perforation are rare, but there are procedural techniques available to help reduce the risk of these complications (discussed later).

*Considering the more common complications of upper endoscopy and knowing that the patient had a stricture dilation, which increases his risk of perforation, you ask for more clinical information about the patient.*

## Is the Fever Associated With Pain?

- Pain is the most common symptom associated with perforation. It may be substernal or pleuritic, depending on the location of the perforation, and may be associated with fever, leukocytosis, and, in some cases, crepitus or a pleural effusion. Other conditions to consider in the setting of fever and pain, particularly with shortness of breath, are aspiration pneumonia and pneumonitis.

- Rarely, chest pain representing myocardial infarction or palpitations representing an arrhythmia may be associated with endoscopy. This is typically an immediate complication rather than delayed.

## Any Change in Voice, Severe Sore Throat, or Neck Swelling?

- Rarely does a tear occur in the upper esophagus or hypopharynx during diagnostic endoscopy.

However, endoscopic dilation or use of an overtube increases this risk. If these symptoms are present, then there is concern for a possible upper para-esophageal or retropharyngeal abscess secondary to perforation.

## Is There Bleeding?

- Bleeding is more common in patients with thrombocytopenia or coagulopathy, but current data suggest that it is rare enough that upper endoscopy is considered safe in patients with platelet counts as low as 20,000. Interventions performed during the procedure, such as endomucosal resection, variceal banding, or ulcer intervention, may increase risk of bleeding or rebleeding.

- Mallory-Weiss tears may occur during or shortly after an upper endoscopy due to retching but are not typically associated with significant bleeding. They occur in fewer than 0.1% of all diagnostic endoscopies.[1]

## What Examination and Studies Should Be Performed?

- Physical exam: Complete physical examination including palpation of upper neck and shoulders for crepitus. If there is neck edema or voice changes, careful inspection of the oropharynx and palpation for neck tenderness should be performed.

- Labs: Complete blood count (CBC) with differential to assess for infection and bleeding, metabolic profile with attention to blood urea nitrogen (BUN)/creatinine (as BUN may be elevated in upper gastrointestinal [GI] bleed), and coagulation studies. Other labs may include arterial blood gas or type and cross, depending on their respiratory status and likelihood of requiring a blood transfusion or surgical procedure. Blood cultures should be obtained in a febrile patient.

- Radiology: Chest posteroanterior/lateral radiograph is the essential first step to evaluate for possible pneumonia or free air. In general, however, plain films are relatively insensitive. If clinical suspicion is high, the yield from plain films may be increased by administration of water-soluble contrast such as diatrizoate meglumine (Gastrografin), and if still unrevealing, a computed tomography (CT) scan is most sensitive. CT should include the chest and, depending upon the location of symptoms and intervention, the neck.
- Endoscopy report
  - It is always important to review the endoscopy report yourself because there are many subtleties that may not be obvious to the emergency room (ER) doctor without expertise in the field.
  - Important things to consider include the following:
    - Ease of intubation: Difficult intubations can be associated with increased risk of upper esophageal, hypopharyngeal, or retropharyngeal perforation or abscess.
    - Dilation method and stricture type:
      - Most centers use either polyvinyl dilators (Savary-Gilliard), which use a push method over an endoscopically placed guidewire, or balloon dilators depending upon the indication. These are considered the safest methods when compared to their predecessors, which were mercury-filled dilators (Maloney) that used a push method without a guidewire.
      - Benign strictures have a lower risk of perforation (approximately 0.4%), while caustic strictures have the highest risk (as high as 17%). Malignant strictures fall somewhere in the middle, with an estimated 10% risk of perforation.
      - There is some evidence to support that using a stepwise graduated sequence of

  dilations is lower risk than using a single, larger dilation.

  □ A few studies have noted higher risk at pressures greater than 11 psi or dilation diameter greater than 15 mm, although sometimes these pressures or sizes are necessary.

*The resident tells you the patient denies pain but appears uncomfortable. Vitals are significant for a temperature of 100.6°F, heart rate (HR) of 102, blood pressure (BP) of 110/78, and O$_2$ saturation of 98% on 2 L nasal cannula. The exam according to the resident is otherwise unremarkable. You review the procedure note and find that the patient had 3 sequential Savary dilations to 14 french for a stricture in the mid-esophagus. This was increased from his prior dilations but the procedure was otherwise uncomplicated. Labs return with a white blood cell (WBC) of 15, normal hematocrit and platelets, and unremarkable metabolic panel. Chest radiograph shows a right lower lobe infiltrate. The patient is admitted to the medical service for treatment of aspiration pneumonia.*

## BLEEDING AFTER COLONOSCOPY

*You are covering the consult pager overnight on a Friday night and receive a call from the ED about a patient who has come in with blood in his stool. The patient is a 55-year-old man with no significant past medical history who had a screening colonoscopy 2 days ago. He was doing well until today when he had a sudden urge to defecate, followed by evacuation of about 200 cc of bright red blood with clots. He initially hoped it would stop, but since the first bowel movement he's had 2 more episodes, each time with more bright red blood. He became light-headed and slightly nauseous, so his wife brought him to the ER for evaluation.*

*The physician in the ED has taken a detailed history and tells you the patient has been taking ibuprofen for the past day for back pain. The patient has a prescription for 600 mg tablets of ibuprofen and took it 3 times yesterday. The ED physician is concerned about a nonsteroidal anti-inflammatory drug (NSAID)-induced ulcer and asks what you think.*

## SOME INITIAL THOUGHTS

- The differential diagnosis in this patient includes a brisk upper GI source such as a gastric or duodenal ulcer, for which he is certainly at risk, or a more distal bleed secondary to NSAID-induced ulcer, arteriovenous malformations, a bleeding diverticulum, or a postpolypectomy bleed.
- Bleeding that causes symptoms of hemodynamic instability should prompt immediate evaluation and intervention.
- Postpolypectomy bleeding typically occurs in the first few days after polyp removal, but has been reported much later. Postpolypectomy bleeding can be classified as immediate or delayed.
- The incidence of postpolypectomy bleeding is 0.2% to 1.8% of cases, but postpolypectomy bleeds account for up to 8% of all lower GI bleeds.[2]
- Immediate, significant hemorrhage after polypectomy is typically due to inadequate hemostasis of the vessels in the polyp.
- Risk factors for immediate bleeding include polyp size, polyp morphology (sessile versus pedunculated), patient comorbidities (renal or cardiac disease), older age, coordination of polyp cutting and electrical current application, and endoscopist experience.
- Delayed polypectomy bleeding typically occurs in the 14 days after the procedure with the mean occurrence 5 to 7 days after polypectomy (when there is a healing ulcer), but case reports have noted bleeding

up to 29 days after polypectomy. Delayed bleeding typically occurs with polyp removal with hot snare cautery.

- Risk factors for delayed bleeding are polyp size and right-sided lesions.[2,3]
- Resuming anticoagulation with warfarin or heparin within 1 week of polypectomy increases the risk of severe bleeding.
- Aspirin and NSAIDs have not been found to be independent risk factors for postpolypectomy bleeding, and while data on IIb/IIIa inhibitors is more limited, clopidogrel also does not appear to be independently associated with bleeding after polypectomy.[3,4]

## Key Points: Postpolypectomy Bleed

- Postpolypectomy bleeding typically presents as painless hematochezia or bright red blood per rectum. It commonly occurs within the first 14 days after polypectomy, with a mean presentation at 5 to 7 days postprocedure.
- Initial therapy is stabilization of the patient with volume resuscitation, transfusions as needed, and correction of any coagulopathy, followed by diagnostic and therapeutic management with colonoscopy with a rapid bowel preparation.
- If the patient is bleeding briskly and is a poor candidate for colonoscopy, he or she should proceed to angiography or a tagged RBC scan with the plan for angiography if the scan is positive.
- Risk factors for postpolypectomy bleeding include polyp size and morphology, and delayed bleeding is more common with right-sided lesions and those removed with hot snare. Patients who resume anticoagulation with warfarin or heparin within a week of polypectomy are at increased risk of bleeding. Clopidogrel is associated with increased risk of bleeding after polypectomy when taken with aspirin or other NSAIDs.

*You tell the ED physician that you are concerned that the patient may have a brisk upper GI bleed from an NSAID-related ulcer or a postpolypectomy bleed requiring endoscopic intervention. Further assessment of the patient is required.*

## WHAT EXAMINATION SHOULD BE PERFORMED?

- Physical exam should include an assessment of volume status, with particular attention to vitals and orthostatic changes. Consider whether the patient has been appropriately volume resuscitated, or if he has continued active bleeding and may benefit from transfusion.
- Nasogastric (NG) lavage may help localize the bleeding source and provide evidence of ongoing bleeding.
- Complete examination including auscultation and careful palpation of the abdomen to assess for tenderness should be performed.

*You ask that the patient be admitted to the intensive care unit (ICU) because there is evidence of hemodynamic instability.*

## WHAT STUDIES SHOULD BE PERFORMED?

- Labs: CBC, prothrombin time (PT)/international normalized ratio (INR)/partial thromboplastin time (PTT), and type and screen (or cross) are standard for any GI bleed. A metabolic profile may alert you to other patient-specific risks; for example, an elevated BUN may suggest upper source, while thrombocytopenia or hypoalbuminemia may suggest liver dysfunction and raise your suspicion for variceal bleed. Basic labs will help determine if the patient should receive a blood transfusion, fresh frozen plasma, vitamin K, or desmopressin.
- Colonoscopy report: Review the report yourself to confirm the location of removed polyps, the

technique of removal (cold versus hot snare cautery) and alternate pathology such as diverticulosis or rectal ulcer. Look at the prior sedation requirements to guide anesthesia needs.

- Imaging: Typically, endoscopy is the preferred method to evaluate the source of GI bleeding. However, assessment of the patient and his or her status should be frequent, and consideration of red cell labeled radionuclide scan and angiography should be considered as first-line interventions in certain situations.
  - In patients with hemodynamic instability and hematochezia that can quickly be volume re-suscitated, emergent EGD should be considered prior to colonoscopy to exclude a brisk upper GI source.
  - In patients who are hemodynamically stable, emergent colonoscopy is recommended as first-line management. Upper endoscopy should be considered if there is concern for an upper source for the bleeding.

*You ask for the labs and review the colonoscopy report, noting the patient had 2 ascending colon polyps and 1 descending colon polyp that were all removed. The proximal 2 polyps were removed with hot snare, and the distal with cold snare. You sus-pect 1 of the 2 proximal polyps is the culprit, due to the increased risk of delayed bleeding with hot snare. The patient did not have diverticulosis or other pathology. In the ED, he is mildly nauseous, but he has no abdominal pain and is not orthostatic. NG lavage was performed and revealed bile. You re-call, however, that in up to 20% of upper GI bleeds, the NG lavage may be negative.*

*The patient is admitted to the ICU. You go to the hospital to evaluate him, with an initial plan for colonoscopy and surgical consult. In making your plan, you consider the following:*

- Bowel preparation: Preparation for an emergent colonoscopy should include 3 to 6 L of a polyethylene glycol-based solution at a rate of 1 to 2 L/hour. The patient may require an antiemetic or an NG tube to improve tolerability.[4]
- Timing: If the patient is hemodynamically stable and has stopped bleeding, then colonoscopy can be performed when stool has become clear liquid.[4]
- Endoscopic options for therapy include cautery, injection of 1:10,000 epinephrine, and hemostasis clips.
  - Choice of method depends on the lesion and the endoscopist.
  - Coagulation with bipolar probe in the right colon has up to a 2.5% risk of perforation, although it still may be a method of choice.[4] Energy delivered depends on pressure placed on the tissue and the size of the area of contact, which depends on the angle of the probe against the mucosa. Energy delivered by argon plasma coagulator, on the other hand, depends on distance from the tissue, duration of energy, and power setting.
- Though the initial plan for this patient is colonoscopy, should he not tolerate the bowel prep and develop more significant bleeding, angiography would remain an option. Radiology may require a tagged red blood cell (RBC) radionuclide scan prior to angiography because it is less invasive.
  - Typically, tagged RBC scan detects bleeding at a rate of 0.1 to 0.5 mL/min, while angiography detects bleeding at a rate of 0.5 to 1 mL/min; however, these rates vary.
  - Angiography is successful in 70% to 90% of GI bleeding cases without major ischemic complications. When angiography was first introduced, the large catheter size used for angiography caused a high rate of bowel infarction, but catheters are now smaller and hemostasis materials such as microcoils are available for more focused intervention.

- ○ Angiography is more successful in the left colon than the right.
- ○ Angiography is indicated for patients who have hemodynamic instability from massive bleeding (versus surgery) or if colonoscopy fails to identify the source of the bleed in a patient with ongoing bleeding.

*The patient starts the bowel prep via the NG tube in the ICU. He remains hemodynamically stable, and initial labs return with hemoglobin of 10, down 3 points from his baseline hemoglobin of 13. He passes moderate amounts of dark blood with clots during the prep and is transfused on the basis of his active bleeding. You are able to perform the colonoscopy and find rapid oozing at the site of his most proximal polypectomy. You place 2 endoscopic clips and achieve good hemostasis. The team taking care of him asks you to review the key points of the case with them.*

---

### Key Points: EGD

- Almost half of procedure-related complications are attributable to physiologic changes associated with sedation.
    - ¤ A patient's past medical history and the anticipated sedation requirements (particularly a long or complicated procedure) can help in assessing risk of cardiopulmonary complications and when an anesthesiologist may be indicated.
    - ¤ The risk of sedation-related complications is significantly greater once a patient reaches an ASA class of 3 or higher, and the patient should have a pre-procedure anesthesia consultation. Patients with an ASA of 1 or 2 should be viewed on a case-by-case basis with consideration of the risk of the procedure.
- Bleeding, infection, and perforation risk depend on both underlying patient characteristics, such as coagulopathy, as well as procedure specifics, such as difficult intubation, aspiration events, biopsies, and the need for dilation.

*(continued)*

---

### Key Points: EGD (continued)

- Stricture dilation carries variable risk of perforation depending on the type of stricture, with caustic strictures having highest risk, followed by malignant strictures, and then benign strictures.
- Perforation may sometimes be detected on plain films, but if suspicion is high and initial films are negative, CT with water-soluble contrast is the most sensitive imaging modality.
- Immediate surgical consultation and broad-spectrum antibiotics are indicated for patients with perforations.

---

# PAIN AND FEVER AFTER COLONOSCOPY

*It's 8 PM on a Tuesday night, and you receive a call from a patient's home via the hospital operator. It's the daughter of a 65-year-old man who had a colonoscopy today and is having significant abdominal pain. She says he didn't want her to call, but she's worried about him because he is having significant pain. She is wondering if this is normal or if she should bring him in for evaluation. She tells you he had a "normal colonoscopy" with removal of 2 polyps.*

Risks of complications of colonoscopy depend on both patient characteristics and characteristics of the procedure. The most common complications are acute or delayed bleeding, perforation, and postpolypectomy coagulation syndrome.

## INITIAL THOUGHTS

Perforation typically presents with significant pain, abdominal distention, fever, and tachycardia immediately during or after the procedure; later symptoms may include leukocytosis, peritoneal signs, hypotension, and sepsis. Perforations tend to occur in the first 6 to 24 hours, but there are case reports of perforations presenting beyond the first 24 hours, so perforation should always be considered on the differential for postcolonoscopy pain.

- Perforation may occur at the site of polypectomy, but also commonly occurs in the sigmoid colon, where the angulation of the rectosigmoid junction, along with the free mobility of this segment of bowel, make it vulnerable to mechanical tear due to pressure from the shaft of the endoscope.
- For patients older than age 75, there is a 4- to 6-fold increased risk of perforation, which is thought to be due to the colon wall weakening with age.[5,6]
- Bleeding may occur immediately after the procedure or may be delayed up to 30 days (the mean time of presentation after the procedure is 5 to 7 days after colonoscopy).[5-7] The overall incidence of bleeding is 0.3% to 6.1% of polypectomies.[5,6] Bleeding, however, does not typically cause pain.
- Postpolypectomy coagulation syndrome typically presents 1 to 5 days after polypectomy with a hot snare. Symptoms include localized abdominal pain, fever, peritoneal signs, and leukocytosis and reflect thermal injury to the submucosa from snare-polypectomy.

## DID THE PATIENT HAVE PAIN IMMEDIATELY AFTER THE PROCEDURE, OR WAS THE PAIN DELAYED?

- Acute complications include perforation and bleeding, but a delay of several hours may suggest subserosal burn or microperforation.

## IS THE PAIN GETTING BETTER?

- Complications of colonoscopy are rare.
  - Overall risk of bleeding or perforation is 0.3%; however, risk of bleeding or perforation after polypectomy occurs at a rate of 2.3%.

o Pain that is improving may be more consistent with bowel distention from air insufflation during the procedure, which improves as air is evacuated, while pain that is worsening may be more worrisome for perforation or postpolypectomy syndrome.

## ARE THERE ASSOCIATED SYMPTOMS?

*The patient's wife reports that the patient had minimal pain immediately following the procedure, but since arriving home, the pain has become increasingly worse. Pain is worse with ambulation and sitting. He complains of chills. He has not had any bleeding. You ask them to come to the ED for evaluation and place a call to the ED so they'll know he's coming. The ED resident asks if there are any studies you'd like them to perform prior to your arrival.*

## WHAT EXAMINATION AND STUDIES SHOULD BE PERFORMED?

- Complete physical examination including auscultation and careful palpation of the abdomen to assess for tenderness should be performed.
- Labs: CBC with differential will be helpful for evaluating for infection, inflammation, bleeding, or thrombocytopenia. If febrile, obtain blood cultures. The patient may also require PT/INR/PTT and type and screen.
- Colonoscopy report: Review the report yourself to confirm the location of removed polyps, the technique of removal (cold versus hot snare), and alternate pathology such as diverticulosis or rectal ulcer. Look at the prior sedation requirements to guide anesthesia needs.
  - o Risks of polypectomy increase depending upon the type of polyp (sessile versus pedunculated), polypectomy snare technique, and use of

cautery and site of polyp. Most complications of perforation or bleed are related to cautery burn, so while there are not randomized prospective trials, retrospective data report lower incidence of complications from cold snare than other techniques.

o Saline or epinephrine lift has been shown to reduce the risk of hemorrhage and decrease depth of thermal injury, particularly for large, right-sided lesions, but does not reduce the risk of perforation.

o Right-sided, sessile polyps are the highest risk for postpolypectomy bleed or perforation. This has been attributed to the thinness of the wall and therefore greater potential for thermal injury to larger vessels in the ascending colon.

o Tattooing-associated complications are rare (0.22%), but tattooing has been shown to cause histological changes at the site, including tissue necrosis and edema, and rarely colon abscess with peritonitis.[2]

• Imaging, if needed, will be based on physical exam and labs results. CT of the abdomen and pelvis is more sensitive than radiographs for detecting perforation. If the index of suspicion for perforation is high, a CT should be performed despite normal chest, upright, and supine radiographs.

*The patient is evaluated by the ER staff and is found to have a temperature of 99.9°F, HR 103, and BP 136/88. His physical exam is reported to you as an ill-appearing man in no acute distress. His abdomen is diffusely tender with localized right-sided rebound and guarding. An abdominal CT reveals thickening of the colonic wall at the hepatic flexure without free air. Surgery was consulted, and they recommended a trial of supportive therapy. The patient will be admitted to the surgical service. In creating your plan, you consider the following:*

---

### *Key Points: Postcolonoscopy Pain*

- It is common to have some abdominal pain and bloating after colonoscopy, but it is difficult to assess a patient's status over the phone. Complications from colonoscopy are rare, but can be severe. Patients should be referred to the ED for a full assessment if there is concern for complication.
- Perforation
  - Typically presents immediately after procedure, but microperforation may not present for 6 to 24 hours.
  - May be seen on radiographs, but CT abdomen is the most sensitive diagnostic test.
  - Keep patient NPO (nothing by mouth), start intravenous (IV) antibiotics, and consult surgery.
  - There is no endoscopic therapy currently supported by the literature.
- Postpolypectomy coagulation syndrome
  - Rare complication of polypectomy with hot snare cautery.
  - Typically occurs 1 to 5 days after the procedure, secondary to transmural burn after polypectomy.
  - May present with fever, localized abdominal pain, and leukocytosis, but imaging does not show perforation.
  - Managed supportively with pain medications. Typically does not require surgical intervention.

---

- Surgery consult should be obtained for all patients with perforation, regardless of size and severity.
- Nonsurgical management may be appropriate for patients with localized peritonitis without sepsis, depending upon the size of perforation and patient comorbidities.
  - Microperforation typically presents within 6 to 24 hours and is characterized by localized pain without diffuse peritoneal signs.
  - Treatment consists of bowel rest, IV antibiotics, and serial abdominal exams.

    o There are no data to support closing microperforations with clips, so management remains supportive, and repeat endoscopy is not indicated.

*Blood cultures are performed and broad-spectrum antibiotics to cover GI flora are started. Over the next 24 hours, he remains afebrile, and his WBC decreases from 12 to 8. His diet is advanced from NPO to clear liquids and then to solids. He is discharged home on hospital day 3 to complete a 14-day course of antibiotics. Repeat CT of the abdomen and pelvis is scheduled on day 14 to ensure resolution of the perforation and lack of abscess formation. He is instructed to return to the hospital if he develops a fever or begins to feel worse.*

## ABDOMINAL DISTENTION AFTER PERCUTANEOUS ENDOSCOPIC GASTROSTOMY TUBE PLACEMENT

*You are covering the inpatient consult service on a Thursday morning and are called by the house staff regarding a 75-year-old woman with a history of stroke who was admitted overnight with fever. She was just discharged from the hospital last week after her stroke, during which time a percutaneous endoscopic gastrostomy (PEG) tube had been placed for swallowing difficulties. She now returns with the fever, and on physical exam her abdomen seems distended and tender, particularly at the site of her PEG. The team started broad-spectrum antibiotics and is concerned that the abdominal pain may be related to the PEG. They are wondering what they should do.*

- Complications from PEG placement can be divided into 3 groups: complications from the upper endoscopy (typically associated with sedation, but includes aspiration, bleeding, and perforation), complications from the procedure itself (including significant pneumoperitoneum, portal and mesenteric gas, and injury to the colon or small bowel or other organs), and postprocedure complications associated with tube use and wound care.

- o Complications from the upper endoscopy, including bleeding, hemorrhage, and esophageal perforation, are typically evident at the time of the endoscopy or shortly thereafter. Serious complications occur in 0.13% of upper endoscopies, with a mortality rate of 0.004%.[1]
- o Complications from the PEG procedure are either apparent early (pneumoperitoneum with peritonitis, portal venous gas) or late.
- o Complications from tube use or wound care may occur anytime, but commonly occur in the days to weeks following the procedure. These may include the following:
  - Peristomal pain
  - Wound infection or abscess formation
  - Necrotizing fasciitis
  - Buried bumper syndrome

*When was the procedure performed? Is there anything unusual about the procedure that may point toward increased risk of certain complications?*

## Important Things to Note on the Procedure Report and Regarding Wound Care

- Did the patient get pre-procedure antibiotics?
  - o Up to 18% of patients who do not receive antibiotics develop wound infections. Antibiotics reduce the risk of infection to 3%.[8]
- Is there anything in the report to suggest the technique had a lapse in sterility?
- Was the skin incision appropriate?

- o Skin incisions of 1 to 2 mm larger than the feeding tube have been associated with lower risk of wound infection.[8]
- Has the site been kept clean and dry since the procedure?
  - o It should have been kept dry with clean dressings.
- Is there excessive tension of the external bumper against the skin?
  - o Tension of the bumper against the skin increases the risk of developing gastric erosions under the internal bumper and over a longer period of time increases the risk of buried bumper syndrome. Loosening the bumper can facilitate healing of any gastric erosion under the bumper.

*The intern tells you that the PEG site was covered with a 2 x 2 gauze dressing and that when they removed it they noted erythema around the site with either purulent drainage or tube feed leaking out. They are unable to see underneath the external bumper to examine the skin and are afraid to move the bumper. You plan to meet him at the bedside to examine the site together.*

## Physical Examination

- Complete physical examination with attention to the abdominal examination should be performed. Often, the PEG site has a small amount of erythema. It should not be particularly tender unless recently placed. The PEG tube should be able to be twirled easily. The current bumper position should be compared with the position noted on the endoscopy report.

### Labs

- Examination should guide whether a CBC or other labs are necessary.

*Imaging*

- A radiograph of the abdomen can be obtained to look for subcutaneous air or PEG displacement using water-soluble contrast through the PEG.
- CT scan of the abdomen and pelvis will be the most definitive study to look for a possible abscess.
- Pneumoperitoneum is common.
  - More than 50% of patients have evidence of pneumoperitoneum after PEG placement, which is thought to be secondary to air escaping the small opening in the stomach during the interval between needle puncture and PEG tube passage from the stomach to the abdominal wall. Typically, it is self-limited, but concern should be raised if it is enlarging or if it is associated with peritoneal signs.

*You meet the intern at the patient's bedside. On exam, the patient is febrile and confused, and her abdomen is distended and tympanic to percussion. There are no notable bowel sounds. You note the external bolster is at 2.5 cm and note that on the original report it was at 4.0 cm at the end of the procedure. The skin is swollen, and you gently loosen the bumper. The incision itself is mildly erythematous, but there is no purulence, and it does not look cellulitic.*

*In formulating your plan, you consider that most complications related to the procedure present close to the time of the procedure. A call 1 week or more after the procedure is more likely related to wound care or tube manipulation.*

Typical complications related to wound care or tube manipulation include the following:
- Peristomal pain, abscess formation, or wound infection
  - These may require a surgery consult for débridement.

- Necrotizing fasciitis and buried bumper syndrome
  - Necrotizing fasciitis is rare, but typically occurs shortly after the procedure. CT is the most sensitive for diagnosis, and emergent surgery consult is required.
  - Buried bumper syndrome typically occurs after approximately 4 months, but may present anywhere from 2 months to several years after PEG placement. It results from excessive tension on the tube, and the internal bumper may become epithelialized. Symptoms include abdominal pain, difficulty infusing tube feeds, and leaking around the tube. Diagnosis is endoscopic, and regardless of symptoms the tube should be removed to prevent impaction and perforation.
- Bleeding and ulceration
  - The most common endoscopic finding in evaluation of PEG patients for GI bleeding is esophagitis.
  - Gastric pressure ulcers may occur either under the internal bumper or on the lesser curve of the stomach opposite the internal bumper. Avoiding excessive traction and avoiding long tips on the internal bumper can minimize these complications. Anti-secretory therapy may not treat these injuries, and changing the PEG may be necessary.
- Gastric outlet obstruction
  - In adults, this is typically secondary to replacement PEGs with balloon anchors. Migration of the balloon into the pylorus or duodenum can cause obstruction, and it can be avoided by using the external bumper to anchor the PEG.
- Ileus and gastroparesis
  - More common in diabetics and if there is a large amount of postprocedure pneumoperitoneum.
  - May be treated with erythromycin.

**Table 13-1.**

## PERCUTANEOUS ENDOSCOPIC GASTROSTOMY REPLACEMENT

| TIME SINCE ORIGINAL | PLAN |
| --- | --- |
| <7 days | Tract is not matured. Do not reinsert a new PEG blindly. The stomach may have separated from the abdominal wall, and you may introduce peritonitis. <br><br> Make the patient NPO, start broad-spectrum antibiotics, and consult surgery if there are signs of peritonitis. |
| >7 days | Tract is likely matured. If the PEG has been out for less than 2 hours, you can insert a replacement blindly. If it has been out for more than 2 hours, you should consider replacing it endoscopically. |

- o Supportive care consists of unclamping the tube for decompression and holding tube feeds for 24 to 48 hours, as with usual care of ileus.
- Dislodgement
  - o Occurs overall in 1.6% to 4.4% of patients, typically if they are confused or combative.[8] Use of an abdominal binder may help avoid dislodgement in high-risk patients.
  - o Replacement plan depends on when the PEG was placed (Table 13-1).
- Leaking
  - o Leaking occurs with an incidence of 1% to 2%.[8]
  - o There is temptation to replace the tube with a larger tube; however, this can cause the tract to enlarge and exacerbate leakage.

- o If leaking begins a short time after the initial PEG placement, consider nutrition, wound healing, and skin breakdown as possible underlying etiologies to address.
- o If leaking begins after the site has been well healed and it appears healthy, removing the PEG for 24 to 48 hours and allowing the tract to partially close may help. In some cases, replacement of the PEG at a new site is necessary. Some patients may have extremely poor nutritional status, and the site may deteriorate.
- Clogging
  - o Clogging occurs in up to 45% of patients.[8]
  - o The best methods for prevention are flushing the tube with 30 to 60 cc of water every 4 hours and avoiding administration of bulking agents (psyllium) through the tube.
  - o A reasonable approach to unclogging a clogged tube is to start by using warm water and then carbonated beverages. A wire should be avoided to reduce the risk of perforating the tube.

*You are concerned about the degree of tenderness and decide to order an abdominal radiograph with injection of gastrografin through the PEG to verify appropriate placement. The radiograph shows appropriate flow of gastrografin through the PEG into the gastric lumen. There is no pneumoperitoneum and no evidence of perforation. The radiograph does note an ileus as the cause of her distention. The intern wonders if it's related to the PEG, and you explain that while postprocedure ileus and gastroparesis are fairly common after PEG placement, it typically occurs because of the manipulation during the procedure. You do note with respect to her recent procedure that they should exclude an aspiration event as the cause of her fever and leukocytosis because she is at an increased risk of aspiration.*

*You recommend to the team that they closely monitor and correct the patient's electrolytes, minimize anticholinergics, and make her NPO. You suggest that instead of placing an NG tube, they simply uncap the PEG for 24 to 48 hours for bowel decompression to a drainage bag. The remainder of her labs are appropriate, and the patient's pain is already improving after loosening the bumper.*

## Key Points: Percutaneous Endoscopic Gastrotomies

- Minor complications from PEG placements are common but are also fairly easy to treat. Most major complications are identified at the time of endoscopy, with the exception of colon perforation, which may not be detected until a PEG is changed many years later.
- Complications that occur after the time of the procedure are typically related to wound care or manipulation of the tube. This includes wound infection or abscess formation, motility problems, parastomal leaking, and tube dislodgement.
  - Rare but serious complications need to be detected early, including infection, erosion of the internal bumper through the gastric wall and into the peritoneum, and necrotizing fasciitis. Imaging with CT can be quite helpful depending on clinical suspicion.
- Serious complications that you should have a low threshold for evaluating include the following: necrotizing fasciitis, perforation (particularly of small bowel and other intra-abdominal organs), and significant pneumoperitoneum. These all warrant expedited surgical consultation for possible laparotomy.

# Endoscopic Retrograde Cholangiopancreatography

*It's a busy Friday afternoon when you receive a call from the surgical intern about a patient who underwent endoscopic retrograde cholangiopancreatography (ERCP) earlier today for choledocholithiasis. The patient is on the schedule for a cholecystectomy tomorrow but is complaining of severe abdominal pain. They have already done a radiograph of the abdomen, which is unremarkable, but they're still wondering if it could be related to the procedure. You quickly generate the following differential of ERCP complications.*

- Pancreatitis
  - Pancreatitis is the most common complication after ERCP. A transient elevation of pancreatic enzymes frequently occurs, but the American Society for Gastrointestinal Endoscopy (ASGE) defines significant pancreatitis as "new or worsened abdominal pain and an amylase that is 3 times the upper limit of normal 24 hours after the procedure, requiring at least 2 days of hospitalization."[9]
  - Incidence is 1% to 7%.[9-11]
  - Risk factors include the following:
    - Patient characteristics: History of ERCP-induced pancreatitis, sphincter of Oddi dysfunction, female gender, younger age (age <60 or 70, depending on the study).
    - Procedure characteristics: Difficult cannulation of the sphincter, sphincterotomy, pancreatic duct opacification, failure to clear stones, balloon dilation of the sphincterotomy site.[12]
- Hemorrhage
  - Hemorrhage is typically related to sphincterotomy and occurs at a rate of 0.76% to 2%.[9] It may occur up to 2 weeks after the procedure, but half

of all cases are diagnosed either at the time of the procedure or in the first 1 to 2 days after the procedure, when the patient produces melena, hematochezia, or hematemesis.

- Risk factors include underlying coagulopathy, use of anticoagulants in the first 72 hours after sphincterotomy, papillary stenosis, presence of ascending cholangitis, and low case volume of the endoscopist.
- Of note, length of incision and aspirin or NSAID use do not predict bleeding.[13]
- Retroperitoneal hemorrhage may occur.

- Perforation
  - Perforation can be categorized into 3 types[14]:
    - Guide-wire induced perforation
    - Periampullary perforation during sphincterotomy
    - Perforation at site remote from the papilla
- Cholangitis
  - The incidence is less than 1%, but the risk of ERCP-induced cholangitis is increased when the procedure is performed for placement of a stent in a malignant stricture, when biliary drainage is incomplete, and in procedures performed to evaluate jaundice. For this reason, given the risk of incomplete drainage, plastic stent placement is recommended in cases of choledocholithiasis where there is incomplete stone extraction.[9]
- Cholecystitis
  - Cholecystitis occurs in 0.2% to 0.5% of all ERCPs and correlates with the presence of stones in the gallbladder and possibly with filling of the gallbladder with contrast.[9]
- Cardiopulmonary complications
  - Rare (<1%), but the leading cause of death from ERCP.[9]
  - Typically attributed to underlying comorbidities or to complications of sedation.

    ○ Includes arrhythmia, aspiration, hypoventilation.
    ○ May be reduced by involving anesthesiologists
      in difficult cases.

*You ask for more information about the patient from the intern and compare it with information from the ERCP report. The intern tells you that she is a 40-year-old woman with no significant medical history who presented with right upper quadrant pain. Ultrasound showed a stone in the common bile duct, and her ERCP was uncomplicated. When she came back up to the floor, she initially seemed well, but about an hour later the nurse called because the patient was complaining of abdominal pain. The ERCP report notes an uncomplicated procedure, although cannulation of the sphincter was difficult secondary to the patient's anatomy. Sphincterotomy was performed, and the duct was swept with a balloon, removing sludge. The intern asks what other studies he should order before you arrive and see the patient.*

- Physical examination: Complete physical examination should be performed including close inspection, auscultation, and palpation of the abdomen.
- Labs: CBC with differential, metabolic profile, liver function panel, and pancreatic enzymes can be helpful in assessing for infection, acidosis, and signs of bleeding, biliary obstruction, or pancreatitis.
- Imaging: If your suspicion for perforation is high, CT will be more sensitive than a radiograph. The diagnosis of pancreatitis, however, can be made based on CBC and clinical exam alone.

*You arrive to interview and examine the patient. She is comfortable, afebrile, and anicteric, but with moderate epigastric tenderness. She has no rebound or peritoneal signs, and your suspicion is low for perforation. You opt to defer further imaging until after labs come back because her exam is most consistent with pancreatitis and is otherwise reassuring. For her initial management, you consider the following:*

- Post-ERCP pancreatitis is managed with bowel rest, IV fluids, and analgesics. She will be closely monitored for fever, leukocytosis, and worsening abdominal pain, which may suggest either more severe pancreatitis or raise suspicion of perforation.
- Antibiotics are indicated if you suspect cholangitis or perforation.

---

### Key Points

- The most common complications from ERCP are pancreatitis, bleeding, infection, and perforation. These are typically managed as follows:
    □ Pancreatitis: NPO, IV fluids, analgesics.
    □ Bleeding: NPO, correct coagulopathies/hold NSAIDs, supportive transfusions, consider endoscopic therapy. Retroperitoneal bleeding can be a rare but serious complication and should be considered on the differential if clinical suspicion is high.
    □ Infection: NPO, IV antibiotics, consider repeat ERCP if there is concern for ongoing biliary obstruction and cholangitis, surgical consult for cholecystitis (rare).
    □ Perforation: NPO, NG tube decompression, surgical consult, IV antibiotics.
- There should be a low threshold for CT in a patient with pain, tachycardia, fever, or leukocytosis to exclude perforation. Perforation at the sphincter may be retroperitoneal, and 20% to 40% of patients with retroperitoneal perforation may require surgical management.[14]

---

## COMPLICATIONS OF OTHER ENDOSCOPIC PROCEDURES

There are complications common to all procedures:
- Cardiopulmonary complications include arrhythmia, hypoxemia, respiratory failure, and aspiration.

Cardiopulmonary and sedation-related complications account overall for approximately 40% of all endoscopic complications. Complex procedures with anticipated long duration or procedures for patients with multiple comorbidities, particularly cardiovascular or pulmonary disease, may benefit from the sedation expertise of an anesthesiologist.

- Infection, perforation, and bleeding risks depend on the specific procedure and underlying patient characteristics, but are in general low, typically around 0.01 to 0.02%.

- Common complications were discussed previously, but there are a few important complications to note with respect to specific procedures:

  o Endoscopic ultrasound: Exposes patients to the same risks as general endoscopy, but because of needle aspiration, increases the risk of procedure-related infection, perforation, and pancreatitis. The risk of infection can be reduced by following ASGE guidelines for antibiotic prophylaxis at the time of the procedure.

  o Endoscopic mucosal resection: Typically performed for early resection of localized gastric and esophageal cancers or for resection of either upper or lower GI lesions. The procedure consists of an injection of saline into the submucosa for a saline lift, followed by endoscopic resection of the lesion. In addition to the typical endoscopy-related complications, bleeding can be quite significant, with incidence ranging from 1.4% to as high as 20%.[15] There is also a 5% risk of perforation depending on the site and size of resection.

  o Colon and esophageal stents: Colon and esophageal stents may be placed for palliation of esophageal or colonic strictures due to malignancy or temporarily placed for bowel prep prior to surgical resection. At the time of the procedure, these patients have a higher risk of perforation than if they were undergoing standard endoscopy. After stent placement, the risk of migration is dependent on the lesion that was stented—extrinsic compressions carry a high risk of migration (and in many cases a stent is not indicated), while intraluminal malignant lesions have a higher risk of tumor invasion and occlusion than migration. The risk of stent occlusion may be reduced by maintaining a strict low-residue diet, but the most important factor in preventing complications is careful selection of candidates prior to the procedure.

# REFERENCES

1. Eisen GM, Baron TH, Dominitz JA, et al; ASGE Standards of Practice Committee. Complications of upper GI endoscopy. *Gastrointest Endosc.* 2003;57(4):411-445.

2. Dominitz JA, Eisen GM, Baron TH, et al; ASGE Standards of Practice Committee. Complications of colonoscopy. *Gastrointest Endosc.* 2002; 55(7):784-793

3. Sorbi D, Norton I, Conio M, Balm R, Zinsmeister A, Gostout CJ. Postpolypectomy lower GI bleeding: descriptive analysis. *Gastrointest Endosc.* 2000;51:690-696.

4. Barnert J, Messmann H. Diagnosis and management of lower gastrointestinal bleeding. *Nat Rev.* 2009;6:637-646.

5. Levin TR, Zhao W, Conell C, et al. Complications of colonoscopy in an integrated health care delivery system. *Ann Intern Med.* 2006;145(12):880-886

6. Rabeneck L, Paszat LF, Hilsden RJ, et al. Bleeding and perforation after outpatient colonoscopy and their risk factors in usual clinical practice. *Gastroenterology.* 2008;135(6):1899-1906.

7. Sawhney MS, Salfiti N, Nelson DB, Lederle FA, Bond JH. Risk factors for severe delayed postpolypectomy bleeding. *Endoscopy.* 2008;40:115-119.

8. Schrag SP, Sharma R, Jaik NP, et al. Complications related to percutaneous endoscopic gastrostomy tubes. A comprehensive clinical review. *J Gastrointest Liver Dis.* 2007;16(4):407-418.

9. Mallery JS, Baron TH, Dominitz JA, et al; ASGE Standards of Practice Committee. Complications of ERCP. *Gastrointest Endosc*. 2003;57(6):633-638.

10. Lieb JG, Draganov P. Early successes and late failures in the prevention of post endoscopic retrograde cholangiopancreatography. *World J Gastroenterol*. 2007;13(26):3567-3574.

11. Ong T, Kohr J, Selamat D, Yeoh K, Ho K. Complications of endoscopic retrograde cholangiography in the post-MRCP era: a tertiary center experience. *World J Gastroenterol*. 2005;11(33):5209-5212.

12. Siegel JH, Veerappan A, Tucker R. Bipolar vs monopolar sphincterotomy: a prospective trial. *Am J Gastroenterol*. 1994;89(10):1827-1830.

13. Freeman ML, Nelson DB, Sherman S, et al. Complications of endoscopic biliary sphincterotomy. *N Engl J Med*. 1996;335(13):909-918.

14. Ruiz-Tovar J, Lobo E, Sanjuanbenito A, Martínez-Molina E. Pneumoretroperitoneum secondary to duodenal perforation after endoscopic retrograde cholangiopancreatography. *Can J Surg*. 2009;52(1):68-69.

15. Shiba M, Higuchi K, Kadouchi K, et al. Risk factors for bleeding after endoscopic mucosal resection. *World J Gastroenterol*. 2005;11(46):7335-7339.

# Financial Disclosures

*Dr. Uri Avissar* has no financial or proprietary interest in the materials presented herein.

*Dr. Wanda P. Blanton* has no financial or proprietary interest in the materials presented herein.

*Dr. Charles M. Bliss Jr.* has no financial or proprietary interest in the materials presented herein.

*Dr. Audrey H. Calderwood* has no financial or proprietary interest in the materials presented herein.

*Dr. Francis A. Farraye* is a consultant for Braintree Labs, Celgene, and Pfizer and is on the advisory board for Centocor, Prometheus, and UCB. He also receives research support from Prometheus.

*Dr. Joseph Feuerstein* has not disclosed any relevant financial relationships.

*Dr. Stephen D. Humm* has no financial or proprietary interest in the materials presented herein.

*Dr. Christopher S. Huang* has no financial or proprietary interest in the materials presented herein.

*Dr. Sujai Jalaj* has no financial or proprietary interest in the materials presented herein.

*Dr. Aarti Kakkar* has no financial or proprietary interest in the materials presented herein.

*Dr. Joann Kwah* has no financial or proprietary interest in the materials presented herein.

*Dr. David R. Lichtenstein* has no financial or proprietary interest in the materials presented herein.

*Dr. Caroline Loeser* has not disclosed any relevant financial relationships.

*Dr. Robert C. Lowe* has no financial or proprietary interest in the materials presented herein.

*Dr. Daniel S. Mishkin* is a consultant for US Endoscopy.

*Dr. David P. Nunes* has not disclosed any relevant financial relationships.

*Dr. Marcos C. Pedrosa* has no financial or proprietary interest in the materials presented herein.

*Dr. Rajeev Prabakaran* has no financial or proprietary interest in the materials presented herein.

*Dr. Ivonne Ramirez* has no financial or proprietary interest in the materials presented herein.

*Dr. Ashraf Saleemuddin* has no financial or proprietary interest in the materials presented herein.

*Dr. Jennifer A. Sinclair* has no financial or proprietary interest in the materials presented herein.

*Dr. Pushpak Taunk* has no financial or proprietary interest in the materials presented herein.

*Dr. Hillary Tompkins* has no financial or proprietary interest in the materials presented herein.

*Dr. Sharmeel K. Wasan* has no financial or proprietary interest in the materials presented herein.

*Dr. M. Michael Wolfe* has not disclosed any relevant financial relationships.

# Index

Printed in the United States
by Baker & Taylor Publisher Services